THE
OUTWARD BOUND®
WILDERNESS
FIRST-AID
Handbook

THE
OUTWARD BOUND®
WILDERNESS
FIRST-AID
Handbook

JEFF ISAAC, PA-C and PETER GOTH, M.D.

Illustrations by Laura Wininger

Lyons & Burford, Publishers

"TO
THOSE IN THE FIELD"

Library of Congress Cataloging-in-Publication Data

Isaac, Jeff.
The outward bound wilderness first-aid handbook / Jeff Isaac and
Peter Goth ; illustrations by Laura Wininger.
p. cm.
Includes index.
ISBN 1-55821-106-3
1. First aid in illness and injury—Handbooks, manuals, etc.
2. Outdoor life—Accidents and injuries—Handbooks, manuals, etc.
I. Goth, Peter. II. Title.
RC88.9.095I82 1991 91-12682
616.02'52—dc20 CIP

Printed in the United States of America

10 9 8

CONTENTS

Why the Outward Bound® Wilderness First Aid Handbook

Hikers, backpackers, campers, fishermen, canoe trippers, climbers and anyone who ventures into wilderness areas of our country can benefit from the information in this practical book.

For thirty years, Outward Bound USA has been running courses for young people and adults in spectacular wilderness and backcountry areas. Over 250,000 people have graduated from Outward Bound courses—29,000 in 1990 alone. The safety of students and staff is of utmost concern and is our most important priority.

With well qualified staff leading tens of thousands of novice outdoorspeople in a variety of wilderness activities in the backcountry, we have had to cope with a wide variety of emergencies, both with our students as well as during our traditional search and rescue missions.

This book has been developed in conjunction with professionals, such as Wilderness Medical Associates, as a practical and useful guide to all those enthusiasts who use our country's wilderness areas. When you can't call 911 to ask for Emergency Medical Services to come to your assistance, the information in this book will increase your competence and confidence in dealing with an emergency.

It is Outward Bound's hope that with the knowledge available in this book you who travel in remote areas will be able to react more confidently in emergency situations, thereby enhancing the enjoyment and personal renewal found in wilderness activities.

John F. Raynolds III
President
Outward Bound USA

ABOUT OUTWARD BOUND®

Outward Bound is the largest and oldest adventure-based educational institution in the world and is a nonprofit, tax-exempt organization. Best known for its ability to build participants' self-confidence and self-reliance, Outward Bound also develops a sense of compassion for others, responsibility to the community, sensitivity to the environment, and leadership skills in individuals from many different backgrounds.

Outward Bound uses challenging activities, primarily in wilderness settings, to teach both adults and young people more about themselves and others, and to help them realize that many of their preconceived limits are self-imposed.

Each Outward Bound course centers around challenging

activities for which extensive technical training is given. Included among more than 600 courses, offered to people fourteen years of age and older, are experiences ranging in diversity from sailing, backpacking, canoeing, sea kayaking, and whitewater rafting to mountain climbing, skiing, dog sledding and even urban experiences. All use the vast majestic wilderness areas of twenty-two states, as well as selected urban environments in nine major U.S. cities. All incorporate traditional Outward Bound elements like map and compass use, orienteering, rock climbing, rappelling, and wilderness camping.

A BRIEF HISTORY

Outward Bound grew out of the need to instill a spiritual tenacity and the will to survive in young British seamen being torpedoed by German U-boats during World War II. From this beginning in 1941, a number of Outward Bound schools were first established in the United Kingdom. The movement soon spread to Europe, Africa, Asia, Australia and North America. Today there are thirty-two Outward Bound schools and centers on five continents.

The first Outward Bound school in the United States was established in 1961 in Colorado. Now there are five U.S. Outward Bound schools: Colorado; Hurricane Island, in Maine; North Carolina; Pacific Crest, in Oregon; and Voyageur, in Minnesota.

Outward Bound has also established a number of urban programs currently operating in Atlanta, Baltimore, Boston, Chicago, Minneapolis, New York City, Los Angeles, San Diego and San Francisco. These urban programs have been specifically designed to address the needs of inner-city youth and the social, cultural and educational problems existing in every large city throughout the country.

SERVING SPECIAL POPULATIONS

A typical Outward Bound course is from 4 to 9 days for adults, and from 3 to 4 weeks for high school and college students. Outward Bound also offers many courses specifically developed to serve the unique requirements of some special populations: troubled youth, substance abusers, people with special medical needs, victims of domestic violence, and Vietnam veterans suffering from post-traumatic stress disorder. At each school, courses incorporating leadership development and wilderness study may be taken for college credit, and there are also specific courses for professional and managerial groups.

SAFETY IN THE WILDERNESS

All Outward Bound instructors are highly skilled and experienced in wilderness adventure. Training includes the latest technical and safety management practices. Outward Bound's enviable safety record reflects the emphasis each school places on ensuring the well-being of students entrusted to its care.

BENEFITS

After an Outward Bound experience, participants discover many positive attributes about themselves. All expect more from themselves. They become confident whereas before they were hesitant. They learn to share, to lead and to follow, and to work together as a group. In safeguarding each other, they form bonds of mutual trust. They discover that many problems can be solved only with the cooperation of all members of a group.

Over the past half-century, research has validated these universally recognized positive effects on personal growth. Outward Bound is well-known for its ability to enhance confidence and interpersonal relationships, and has been shown to provide marked improvements in many other areas of personal and moral development such as self-esteem, assertiveness, and dependability.

As one Outward Bound student said: "We are better than we know. If we can be made to see it, perhaps for the rest of our lives we will be unwilling to settle for less."

For further information, please call or write Outward Bound USA, 384 Field Point Road, Greenwich, CT 06830, (203) 661-0797 or toll-free (800) 243-8520.

PREFACE

Outward Bound is a worldwide system of schools that operates educational programs in a wilderness setting. Outward Bound has always been committed to the highest standards of safety and has long been a leader in developing safety standards in outdoor education. Outward Bound also has a commitment to public service. Rescue and emergency response have been a traditional service component of the Outward Bound program—most Outward Bound schools have an active search and rescue (SAR) team and regularly work with professional medical teams to locate, access, stabilize and transport missing and injured persons.

For years, backcountry enthusiasts, outdoor schools, wilderness guides, and park rangers went out in the woods armed with first-aid training, techniques and philosophies that were developed for use in the city. It was obvious that new and more appropriate principles and procedures for backcountry first-aid were needed. Some just accepted it as the way things were. Others, like Outward Bound, knew there had to be a better way and went looking for it. This book was written in the hope that some of the principles, approaches and perspectives regarding backcountry emergency care that are used by Outward

Bound staff can be shared with the public.

Conventional first-aid training programs and instructional texts are designed for an urban or suburban context and generally assume that conventional medical resources are readily available. The Emergency Medical Services (EMS) system that is activated by a 911 call is in fact built upon the concept of a "Golden Hour." The experience of military medics and MASH units in Korea and Viet Nam taught the important lesson that the likelihood of survival is greatly enhanced if a patient is delivered to the operating room within an hour of the initial injury. As a result, most first-aid books and training emphasize that your best treatment is stabilization and rapid delivery to the hospital emergency room.

Special problems occur when medical care is required in a backcountry setting. For these illnesses and injuries, rapid transport is usually not an option. "Wilderness medicine" is a specialized approach to field medical care that represents some new and exciting concepts. It specifically addresses the special and unusual kinds of medical problems that occur in a backcountry setting. New approaches to field medical treatment are often required for "off road" emergency situations. These situations often involve extended or delayed patient transport, prolonged management of illnesses and injuries, and the need to deal with medical emergencies in a remote field setting, far away from the easy access of 911, hospitals and the usual medical resources of civilization. The wilderness context often is further complicated by severe environments and the need to rely on limited or improvised equipment.

Today, wilderness medicine is a "specialty." Physician groups such as the Wilderness Medical Society regularly conduct special research projects and conferences on backcountry medical problems. Non-profit organizations such as the National Association for Search and Rescue (NASAR) conduct and certify specialized wilderness-medical training programs across the country. Most Outward Bound instructors, park rangers, river guides and others now use medical training programs designed especially for the backcountry. The creation of this book is the result of a collaboration between the leading source of outdoor education, Outward Bound, and the leading source of backcountry medical training, Wilderness Medical Associates, Inc.

Outward Bound was instrumental in the development of new programs and new professional standards in wilderness emergency care. Initial prototypes of the nationally certified NASAR Wilderness Medicine Programs were actually developed and conducted especially for Outward Bound instructors in 1984 by Dr. Peter Goth and Wilderness Medical Associates consulting group. Today, most Outward Bound instructors in the USA are trained and certified according to the NASAR wilderness medicine training curricula. The content of this book reflects the medical training which these Outward Bound instructors have received.

Today, there is an obvious trend toward increasing use of the backcountry for recreation and education. The good news is that more people are exposed to the spectacular beauty and experiences that nature has to offer. The bad news is that more people get sick or injured in backcountry situations, far from conventional medical resources. They often have to rely on their own ingenuity and luck, and there seems to be an ever increasing need to share some of the concepts of wilderness medicine that have been developed for professional use. Hikers, campers, canoe trippers, fishermen, climbers, and others all have a serious need for this information.

This book is intended to provide information which is not only useful, but is also understandable. We have attempted to go beyond the "laundry lists" of signs, symptoms and treatment plans (if you see A and B, do C and D but never do E unless you see F first) which are both confusing and all too common in first-aid books. Instead, we want the reader to understand why problems happen, how to recognize both the obvious and the subtle clues the body gives to reveal its condition, and how to devise and implement practical, flexible and effective treatment plans. The wilderness medicine training programs that were originally developed for Outward

Bound staff reflect a new approach. They are an innovative way of thinking and reacting to any medical emergency, but have special application to the remote backcountry setting where help is far away.

This book is intended to share this approach with others. We first help you to understand how the normal, health body functions; then we can look at the changes in those normal functions which occur with an illness or injury. This information allows us to understand the actual mechanism of what goes wrong and leads to the problem. The next step is to learn how to assess the problem; we offer the same techniques your doctor uses: gather and review all of the information available, analyze it in light of what you know about how things are supposed to work, and finally, make a reasonable diagnosis based on the information you are presented with. The final link in the sequence is to devise a treatment plan based on your diagnosis; we offer concise and practical advice on how to manage most problems. We also add a sophisticated emphasis—monitoring the condition of your patient and continuing to review the clues which leader to your assessment of the injury. Over time, it is likely that these will change, and so will your treatment plan.

Finally, the reader should note that this book is *not* meant to be a comprehensive medical text; it is simply intended to share some of the perspectives, methods and techniques for managing a variety of medical problems in the specialized backcountry context. These have been helpful to Outward Bound and our intention is that they can possibly help others who might need it for their own personal use on their own personal adventures. Those who wish to develop further knowledge and experience and to pursue further training should contact:

Wilderness Medical Associates (WMA)
RFD 2 Box 890
Bryant Pond, ME 04219
207-665-2707

DISCLAIMER

The information contained in this book is intended to serve as a guide for those who may need to provide first aid. It is not intended to be a substitute for professional medical advice or training. The authors disclaim any responsibility or liability for any loss that may occur as a result of information, procedures or techniques included in this work. *Few would venture into the woods not knowing how to pitch a tent or light a stove—first-aid training is equally essential knowledge and should be an integral part of all trip planning.*

A NOTE ON THE ➡ "TREATMENT" SYMBOL

We have added the ➡ arrow to help you quickly pinpoint specific treatments for the medical problems discussed in this book. This has been done to save time in an emergency. Remember, however, that no treatment can be completely effective without a thorough knowledge of the overall issues. We recommend close reading, at home, of the entire text before attempting any wilderness first-aid procedures.

ACKNOWLEDGEMENTS

This book represents the collective wisdom of literally hundreds of people. It is the result of a basic idea which has been subjected to years of refinement, revision and elaboration. Our appreciation and thanks are extended to all of those individuals and organizations who participated in and contributed to our programs over the years.

In particular, we would like to thank the Instructors, Course Directors and Program Directors of Outward Bound for all their comments, suggestions, ideas, solutions to problems and advice which was thoughtfully and freely given. The Sugarloaf Mountain Ski Patrol has provided a depth of resources which would be hard to equal. Lewis Glenn took the time to carefully review the manuscript and offer cogent advice on improvement. Laura Wininger was incredibly patient and persevering in her efforts to develop the drawings which illustrate this book so well. The National Association for Search and Rescue (NASAR) deserves special mention and thanks for its commitment and support for the establishment of national standards for wilderness medical training programs.

Finally, this book could not have been written without the support of Wilderness Medical Associates. Its theories, philosophies, training programs and course materials form the foundation upon which this book rests. Our heartfelt thanks go to the WMA staff—David Johnson, Jim Morrissey, Paul Marcolini and Reid and Ted Forbes—who managed the project, critiqued the manuscript and provided moral support.

Jeff Isaac, PA-C,
Peter Goth, M.D.

INTRODUCTION

The expedition is over and my students are returning to life ashore, some reluctantly, some delighted to be back. Personally, I'm looking forward to some time on my own. Teaching an Outward Bound course is an exercise in perpetual responsibility. While I accept it gladly, I surrender it equally enthusiastically when the time comes. Now I have an appointment with 14 miles of upcountry whitewater.

The back of my pickup is packed with wetsuits, gloves, piles of polypropylene and the rest of the paraphernalia associated with spring paddling in Maine. Crowning the heap is my battered canoe. Her scars are a cumulative history of all of the rocks, stumps, and other boats we've encountered over the years. In reality she is damaged equipment. But, in spirit she is a symbol of both the joys and misery of my encounters with the river.

My own bumps, bruises and scars have healed. Fortunately, all were minor. But, if they weren't, I hope that I'd view them with the same degree of respect and acceptance. Risk is part of the game, and injury can be one of the consequences.

This weekend thousands of paddlers will overturn their boats, climbers will fall, and hikers will become lost. The perceived risk involved in this is usually much greater than the actual danger. This is certainly true in the carefully controlled environment of an Outward Bound program.

Nevertheless, most of us understand that in many worthwhile activities there are real dangers. In Outward Bound courses, we strive to balance these dangers against the joys and benefits of intimate experience with wild country and natural forces. This is the sensitive balance known as "acceptable risk."

Hazards are not sought for their own sake, but neither are they completely avoided. For backcountry travelers, an important part of striking the balance is preparation for handling dangerous situations when they occur. This includes a logical, common sense approach to personal injury which takes into account all aspects of the environment in which we are operating.

In our "civilized" settings we delegate this responsibility to trained professionals. It is the business of paramedics, nurses, P.A.'s and M.D.'s to recognize medical emergencies and know what to do about them. This system allows everyone else to get by with knowing only immediate and temporary treatments, and still keep the risk of daily living within the range of "acceptable."

But once you leave the civilized world behind, the situation changes dramatically. Techniques and equipment developed for the emergency room or ambulance are often inappropriate or impossible outside of the hospital setting. In most wilderness scenarios, a team of sled dogs would be more useful than a team of surgeons.

Getting an injured person out to civilized medical care is

rarely easy. Even when performed by skilled rescuers, a backcountry evacuation is difficult, expensive, and often hazardous. The popular television image of helicopters swooping to the rescue bears little resemblance to reality. Even where available, safe helicopter operation is limited to a fairly narrow range of weather and terrain conditions. The "heroic" rescue is usually an arduous, sweaty, muddy scramble that disrupts the lives of dozens of people.

The object, therefore, in preparing for backcountry medical problems is not to find more and better ways to scream for help, or to stuff your pack with specialty first-aid kits. It is to develop a good basic understanding of the body's structure and functions, and to learn some basic techniques for preserving these functions in the presence of injury. These are the goals of this books.

It is, of course, important to recognize that there are considerable limits to your ability to affect the outcome of some medical emergencies. There are times when screaming for help is absolutely the right thing to do. And there are times when all the help in the world won't make any difference. The vast majority of situations, however, are well within the capabilities of every backcountry traveler to handle.

Like all things remote from civilization, wilderness medicine is elemental. The most important skill is improvisation, and good improvisation requires a solid understanding of the principals behind the treatment. It's a skill like reading a river. The technical information is important, but it's the gut feeling for the subject that gets you through.

We have arranged the material in this book to emphasize this concept. We start by covering generic principals which are common to all injury and illness, and outlining a system for organizing your response. After developing a general level of understanding, we talk about some of the most common specific problems you might encounter.

In each topic, the path to effective treatment begins with understanding the *Mechanism of Injury.* This refers to the cause of the problem at the anatomic level. For example: the mechanism of injury for a broken leg could be a brief foot entrapment in a violent rapid. The mechanism of injury for nerve damage could be nerve entrapment by displaced bone fragments in a broken leg.

The next step is *Assessment*, which is the process of identifying the problems and their relative severity. For example: leg fractures are associated with a positive mechanism of injury followed by pain, deformity, and tenderness. Nerve impairment is revealed by loss by sensation in an injured extremity.

The goal is effective *Treatment.* You can already see that stabilizing and realigning the fragments of a leg fracture would be the best way to prevent nerve damage and other long-term disability.

Sometimes the principles and procedures are quite specific, such as in the management of a dislocated shoulder, or the treatment of an allergic reaction. More often, though, they are general in nature and adaptable to a variety of situations.

We hope that this format will succeed in sharing some of our experience with you. We also hope to stimulate your interest in further education, and greater competence and self-sufficiency in the wilderness. You are, after all is said and written, your own responsibility.

THE
APPROACH
TO
MEDICAL
PROBLEMS

1

ORGANIZED THINKING

Problems, by their very definition, imply a state of instability. Any problem-solving situation can be improved by the use of an organizational technique that frames the unstable problem within a stable system. In other words, trying to impose order on chaos.

In the hospital emergency-department setting, clear priorities are established whereby the most life-threatening conditions are dealt with first, even though a specific diagnosis is often unavailable. What occurs is a generic process of stabilizing and supporting the vital functions of the Circulatory, Respiratory, and Nervous Systems. These "BIG 3" body systems include the most important and sensitive organs—heart, lungs, brain and spinal cord. They constitute the critical machinery most essential to life. Only after the immediate threats to the patient's life have been stabilized, can the process of more specific diagnosis and treatment begin.

The same principle is followed in the backcountry setting. However, because we have only basic diagnostic equipment (our hands, eyes, and ears) and limited options for treatment, the medical problems and treatment plans remain general in nature. Bear in mind that these limits are imposed by the environment, not your training or intelligence.

This makes things a whole lot easier from a medical point of view. For example, you don't need to memorize twelve different causes of abdominal pain, you only need to know when to consider abdominal pain potentially serious. Even if you could distinguish an acute appendicitis from a perforating ulcer, you're not going to haul out your Swiss Army knife and operate on either one.

Remember also, in the hospital emergency department the patient's medical problem is the only thing the doctor needs to worry about. He or she is working in a stable environment with the resources and time to focus on specific medical problems. In the backcountry, however, the patient's medical problem is only a small part of a much larger picture which includes weather, terrain, the condition of the group, available assistance, and a number of other factors.

You will very likely be caring for an injured partner for hours or days. Your plan needs to address not only problems that exist immediately, but problems which can develop later. All of these additional factors reinforce the need to keep the medical part of the response simple and generic.

THE PATIENT ASSESSMENT SYSTEM
(PAS)

In the pre-hospital and backcountry setting the main tool for organized response is the *Patient Assessment System* (PAS). The PAS is based on information gathered in a series of sur-

veys, and organized in a standard format abbreviated "SOAP."
It consists of three important steps: gathering information, organizing a response, and anticipating problems which may develop over time.

GATHERING INFORMATION—SURVEYS

1. SCENE SURVEY
2. PRIMARY SURVEY
3. SECONDARY SURVEY

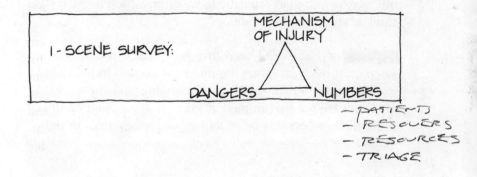

1 - SCENE SURVEY:

MECHANISM OF INJURY

DANGERS — NUMBERS

— PATIENTS
— RESCUERS
— RESOURCES
— TRIAGE

1. SCENE SURVEY

Danger to Rescuers and Patient: Before rushing to the rescue, be sure that you are not going to become another casualty. You can't help anybody else if you're out of commission yourself. It can take tremendous discipline to overcome the powerful urge to come to the immediate aid of a friend in trouble. But this is exactly what you must do, at least for the moment. Stop, look around, and ask yourself: "what's trying to kill me?" It may be frigid water, another avalanche, or more wasps in the nest. Whatever it is, if it can disable you it must be stabilized before you can do anything else.

Once you are safe, or relatively so, look for any further threat to the injured person: "what's trying to kill him?" Stabilize the scene by moving danger from the patient, or the patient from the danger. This has priority over everything else that follows. So, get the patient out of the water, out from under the cornice, or away from the wasps before proceeding with evaluation and treatment.

Mechanism of Injury: Another important element in the survey of the scene is determining the mechanism—or cause—of injury. This may be pretty obvious, but occasionally more investigation will be necessary. For example, how far did he fall? Was it enough of a tumble to cause injury? Are there other factors, such as exposure to weather, which might be the cause of the patient's condition?

Number of Patients: Determine how many people are injured or at risk. Casualties are often overlooked in the rush to treat the most obvious and uncomfortable problems. This is especially true of environmental injuries where most or all expedition members can be in danger of hypothermia or dehydration.

2. PRIMARY SURVEY

This is the initial patient examination. You are checking the status of the BIG 3 systems, looking only for conditions

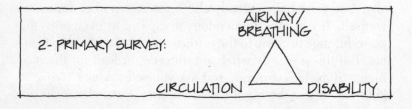

which represent an immediate threat to life. Check to be sure that the mouth and nose are clear to allow the passage of air, and that air is actually going in and out. Observe that blood is circulating and not running out all over the ground. Finally ensure that the patient's spine is stable and that the central nervous system is functioning normally. This is checking the "ABCD's":

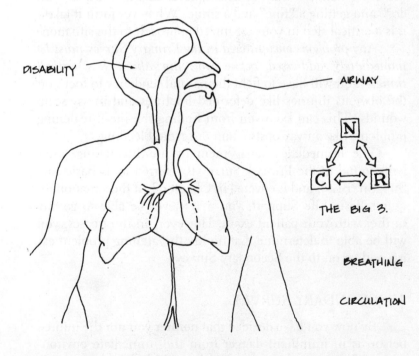

DISABILITY

AIRWAY

N

C ⟷ R

THE BIG 3.

BREATHING

CIRCULATION

A—Airway   – Nose and Mouth > **RESPIRATORY**
                Clear   **SYSTEM**
B—Breathing   – Air moving in   > **RESPIRATORY**
                and out   **SYSTEM**
C—Circulation – Check for Pulse > **CIRCULATORY**
                                 SYSTEM
              – Severe Bleeding > **CIRCULATORY**
                                 SYSTEM
D—Disability – Spine Stable   > **NERVOUS SYSTEM**
              – Level of   > **NERVOUS SYSTEM**
                Consciousness

Performing a Primary Survey may mean hanging upside down in a crevasse listening for breath sounds in your unconscious partner, and feeling inside bulky clothing for blood. On the other hand, it may be as simple as asking "how do you do?" and getting a "fine" and a smile. Whatever form it takes, it is a critical step in your organized approach to the situation.

Any problems encountered in the Primary Survey must be immediately addressed before worrying about less critical things. You will have to fight the natural tendency to focus on the obvious injuries like deformed fractures and messy scalp wounds. This can keep you from finding the life-threatening problems like airway obstruction or severe bleeding.

The immediate management of life-threatening problems found in the Primary Survey is referred to as Basic Life Support (BLS), and is covered in Chapter 3. If the situation requires Basic Life Support, you may never be able to go any further with your patient exam. However, in most cases, you will be able to determine that no life-threatening problem exists and go on to the Secondary Survey.

3. SECONDARY SURVEY

By now you have decided that neither you nor the injured person is in imminent danger from the immediate environment. The patient has no medical problems which are going to kill him or her right now. The scene is stable. The patient is stable.

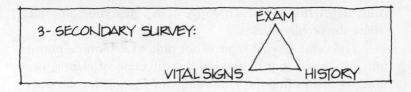

3- SECONDARY SURVEY:

EXAM

VITAL SIGNS   HISTORY

Exam: This stage is a slower, more deliberate examination of the whole patient. It is less urgent than the primary survey, but speed and detail change with circumstances. Unless your primary survey missed something, it is not necessary or efficient to stop and treat problems as you find them. Complete your list, then return to treat later in order of priority.

Although it really makes no difference in what order you proceed, most examiners like to start with the head and neck, moving to the chest, abdomen, pelvis, back, legs, and arms. You are looking, touching, and feeling for abnormality, that is, tenderness (pain caused by touch), swelling, deformity, discoloration, or bleeding. You should be gentle, moving the patient as little as possible. Your exam should be as comprehensive as the situation allows. In the backcountry setting, you don't need mystery and surprises. Touch and look at everything.

Vital Signs: These measurements provide another way of assessing the function of the BIG 3 body systems. The major parts of the Circulatory, Respiratory, and Nervous systems are hidden from our view. We need to rely on indirect methods of watching them work.

Vital signs are like the gauges on the dashboard of your car. Every time you drive you are looking at the same standard gauges; oil pressure, charge indicator, and engine temperature. You can evaluate the health of your car without opening the hood and taking the engine apart. You might not know what the exact readings are supposed to be, but you'll certainly notice if the reading is different from what it usually is. They serve to draw your attention to any deviation from normal.

And, depending on which gauge it is, give you some idea where the problem lies.

The value of vital signs is not only to determine normal from abnormal, but to observe the direction of change over time. By measuring the same standard signs at regular intervals, you can get a sense for improvement or decay in a patient's condition. Is your treatment working? Are things getting better or worse? Is it time to panic, or sit back and have another handful of gorp?

The detail with which you measure vital signs will depend on the equipment available. Vital signs are listed below, with the range of normal values in parentheses.

VITAL SIGNS

T: **Time** when vital signs are measured
BP: **Blood Pressure** in mm of mercury (140/90–110/60)
P: **Pulse** in beats per minute (60–100)
R: **Respiratory rate** in breaths per minute (12–18)
C: **Consciousness** and mental status (AVPU)
T: **Temperature** of the body core (97.6 F–99.6 F)
S: **Skin** color, temperature, moisture

Now, if you'd rather devote the precious space in your pack to peanuts and M&M's instead of blood-pressure cuffs, stethoscopes, and clinical thermometers, you're not alone. Even if a watch is too much technology for you, a valuable assessment of vital signs can still be made. Measurements become relative, for example pulse is "fast" or "slow," temperature is "cool" or "warm." Blood pressure can be assessed as "normal" or "low" based on signs of adequate or inadequate blood flow (more on that later).

Level of Consciousness (C) is a measure of Nervous System (brain) function. No special instruments are required. Consciousness is described as relating to one of four letters on the "AVPU" scale:

AVPU SCALE

A—Alert.
V—responsive to Verbal stimulus.
P—responsive only to Painful stimulus.
U—Unresponsive to any stimulus.

This is a widely used and relatively precise description which avoids confusing terms such as "semi-conscious" and "in and out." Alert patients (A on AVPU) are further described by their mental status. This refers to the patient's level of orientation and anxiety. People with normal mental status generally know who they are, where they are, what day it is, and why they're here. You'll have to allow some slack for time in the woods, of course. We've had perfectly healthy Outward Bound students on long expeditions unable to keep track of the month, never mind the day of the week.

History: The final act in the process of gathering information is to obtain a relevant History. The acronym for what to ask is abbreviated "AMPLE":

HISTORY ASSESSMENT

A—**Allergies:** to insect stings, foods, medications, etc.
M—**Medication:** that the patient is currently taking
P—**Past History:** of similar or related problems
L—**Last Meal:** time and content of last meal
E—**Events:** events leading up to the incident

Of course, we realize that the entire Primary and Secondary Survey may not always be necessary. A simple laceration of the finger by a knife blade while slicing an apple doesn't warrant a full body examination. However, many accident scenarios are unwitnessed, confused by pain and anxiety, and involve hidden injuries. Even in a very straightforward situation, your own level of anxiety as a rescuer may require that you have a structure to function within. An orderly system will do a lot to put your mind at ease and stabilize an uncomfortable situation.

ORGANIZING YOUR RESPONSE—SOAP

The system of organization commonly used by the medical profession is the "SOAP" format. SOAP is the acronym for *Subjective, Objective, Assessment,* and *Plan.* It is a simple and effective management process from the gathering of information, through the identification of the problems, to the formation of a plan to deal with each problem. It is the way medical records are written, and the order in which medical information is communicated. The general meaning of each heading is as follows:

SOAP:	S - SUBJECTIVE O - OBJECTIVE A - ASSESSMENT (A' - ANTICIPATED PROBLEMS) P - PLAN

S—**Subjective:** What happened? Where does it hurt? Relevant history.

O—**Objective:** Information gathered by observation and examination. Include vital signs.

A—**Assessment:** Based on the subjective and objective findings, what is the problem? If more than one, list in order of priority.

P—**Plan:** What are you going to do about each problem now?

Using this system, a typical brief SOAP for an emergency-room case might look like this:

S: A 9-year-old boy fell off his bicycle. He complains of pain in his right wrist and tingling of his fingers. He has no complaints of pain anywhere else.

O: An alert, oriented but uncomfortable boy. The right wrist is swollen and tender to touch. The patient refuses to move the wrist voluntarily. The fingers are warm and pink and can be wiggled with slight pain felt at the wrist. The patient can feel the light touch of a cotton swab on the end of each finger. The boy has no other apparent injuries.

A: Fracture of the right wrist.

P: Splint wrist. Follow up with an orthopedic surgeon in three days. Return to the hospital if fingers become blue or cold, or the tingling becomes at all worse.

This format paints a nice picture of the situation. You get a sense for who the patient is, what happened, how he got to the E.R., and what the physician is going to do about it. There is also a brief description of problems which might occur, and what the response should be.

The SOAP format is perfectly adaptable to the backcountry setting, and it performs the same vital function that it does in the hospital. It organizes your thoughts, renders order from chaos, and allows you to communicate your ideas and plans.

But, we need to expand SOAP a little to take into account the environment in which we are traveling. We must consider problems created by weather, terrain, distance, and time. These factors are just as important to our planning as the condition of the patient.

In long-term care, which describes most backcountry scenarios, we add a section called "**Anticipated Problems**" (**A'**).

This is a list of problems which may develop over time. They could be complications of the injury itself, or the potential result of exposure to environmental factors. By including **A'** in the SOAP note we are in a better position to prevent problems from developing, and be ready to deal with them when they can't be avoided.

```
┌─────────────────────────────────────────────────────┐
│  MONITOR:    REPEAT SURVEYS                          │
│              LOOK FOR A'                             │
│              REVISE SOAP                             │
└─────────────────────────────────────────────────────┘
```

WATCHING FOR CHANGE—MONITOR

As your patient's condition, the weather, and your logistical situation all change with time, plans will need to be revised. The best organizational method for doing this is to repeat the relevant parts of your surveys, and revise your SOAP at regular intervals. This is where you watch for the Anticipated Problems (A') you've listed in your original SOAP note.

Patients with potential BIG 3 problems should be reevaluated most often, at least every fifteen minutes if possible. The CSM (Circulation, Sensation, Movement) of injured extremities can be checked less frequently at one or two-hour intervals. Conditions which develop slowly, such as wound infection, might be adequately monitored every six hours.

With these specialized additions to SOAP in mind, let's take that previous case into the back country:

S: A nine-year-old boy fell onto his outstretched right arm while gathering wood near the Speck Pond Shelter.

He complains of pain in his right wrist and tingling of his fingers. He has no complaints of pain anywhere else. He does not feel cold or hungry. He is known not to have allergies, be on medication, or have any significant medical problems. He had just finished a snack. The fall was due to slipping on wet leaves, and not from a significant height.

It is now sunset. The air temperature is 60 degrees. It is raining lightly.

O: An alert, responsive but uncomfortable boy is found sitting on a rock holding his right arm. He is warm, dry and adequately dressed. His right wrist is slightly swollen and tender to touch. He can wiggle his fingers and feel the light touch of the examiner's hand. His skin color is normal. There is no other injury.

A: Fracture of the right wrist.

A': 1. Swelling and ischemia (inadequate blood flow to the extremity)
2. Difficult hike out

P: 1. Splint the wrist, keep the patient quiet and the arm elevated.
2. Monitor CSM right hand every hour, adjust the splint if necessary.
3. Camp here tonight, walk out in daylight tomorrow.

Even in more complicated cases where a patient may have more than one problem, the format remains the same. Under A (Assessment) we would list the problems in order of priority, and be sure that we have a plan for each one. By checking each problem for a plan, and each plan for a problem, we can avoid missing anything. We can also avoid the very human practice of making plans for problems that don't exist.

PAS - SUMMARY

GATHERING INFORMATION - SURVEYS

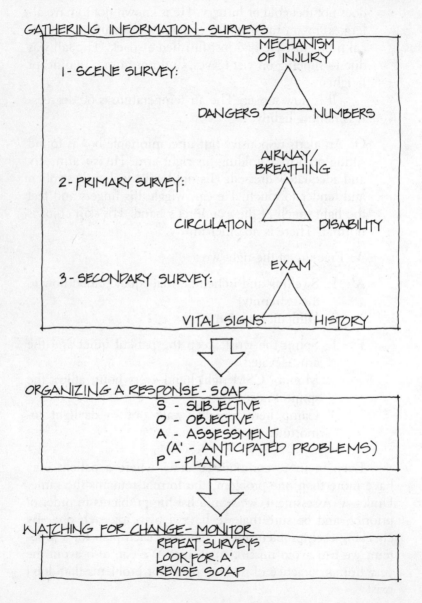

1 - SCENE SURVEY:

MECHANISM OF INJURY

DANGERS   NUMBERS

2 - PRIMARY SURVEY:

AIRWAY/ BREATHING

CIRCULATION   DISABILITY

3 - SECONDARY SURVEY:

EXAM

VITAL SIGNS   HISTORY

ORGANIZING A RESPONSE - SOAP

```
S - SUBJECTIVE
O - OBJECTIVE
A - ASSESSMENT
 (A' - ANTICIPATED PROBLEMS)
P - PLAN
```

WATCHING FOR CHANGE - MONITOR

```
REPEAT SURVEYS
LOOK FOR A'
REVISE SOAP
```

2

GENERAL PRINCIPLES
OF WILDERNESS MEDICINE

Simply memorizing treatment procedures, or carrying a set of flash cards in your pocket, is far from acceptable preparation for medical emergencies. Unless you frequently use or practice memorized procedures, you will forget them. Your instruction card will never be there when you need it, and you won't have time to read it anyway.

Practical preparation for medical emergencies involves truly understanding the principles behind the procedures. If you can accomplish this, you will never "forget" what to do— you will *understand* what needs to be done. Your response may not be in the exact order detailed by the various written protocols, but it will be as appropriate and effective as the situation allows.

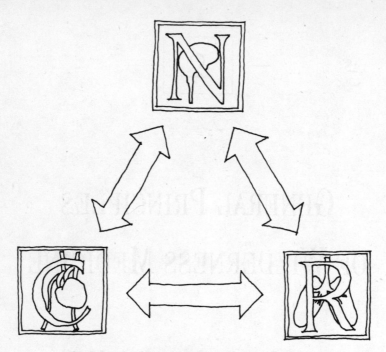

The Big 3 body systems: Circulatory, Respiratory, and Nervous Systems.

THE BIG 3 BODY SYSTEMS

Injury or illness which is life threatening involves a major problem with the Circulatory, Respiratory, or Nervous Systems (BIG 3). These three systems exist in an interconnected triad. Problems with one are quickly reflected in the other two. For example, serious respiratory problems, such as asthma, produce an increased heart rate (Circulatory system) and changes in mental status and consciousness (Nervous system). If any of the BIG 3 actually stop functioning, death occurs within a matter of minutes.

The vital organs of these BIG 3 systems are contained within the BIG 3 body cavities—the head, chest, and abdomen. These organs are not generally accessible to direct exam-

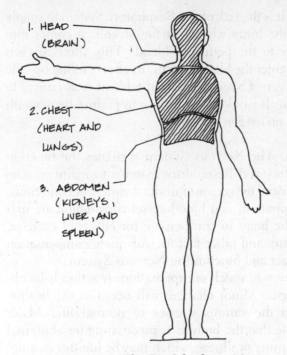

1. HEAD
   (BRAIN)

2. CHEST
   (HEART AND
   LUNGS)

3. ABDOMEN
   (KIDNEYS,
   LIVER, AND
   SPLEEN)

The Big 3 body cavities

ination. We must use indirect signs and symptoms to assess the status of the BIG 3 systems.

Perfusion: The function of the Circulatory System is to force blood through the beds of tiny blood vessels, called capillaries, in all body tissues. This brings blood in close proximity to living cells to allow oxygen, nutrients, and waste to be exchanged between the cells and the blood stream. This is "perfusion," and it is essential to any living tissue.

Considerable pressure is required to push the blood through the capillary beds. This "perfusion pressure" (blood pressure) is generated by the pumping action of the heart, balanced by the ability of the larger blood vessels to constrict. Adequate perfusion requires adequate pressure.

Oxygenation: It is the task of the Respiratory System to supply outside air to the lungs where, in the alveoli, it comes into close proximity to the perfusing blood. This allows oxygen from the air to enter the blood stream, in effect "filling up" the blood with oxygen. Oxygenation of the blood is as critical to life as perfusion. It would be of no use to perfuse tissues with blood that had no oxygen to deliver.

Compensation: The Nervous System regulates the function of the Circulatory and Respiratory Systems to maintain adequate perfusion and oxygenation under a variety of conditions. Heart rate, respiration, and blood-vessel constriction are manipulated by the brain to compensate for effects of exercise, cold, heat, injury and other factors. Adequate compensation requires an intact and functioning Nervous System.

The best way to watch compensation in action is by observing vital signs. Minor changes will occur as the healthy body adapts to the various stresses of normal life. Major changes indicate that the body is compensating for abnormal stress, such as injury or illness, which may be life-threatening.

Shell/Core Effect: One of the primary compensation mechanisms seen in stress and injury is the shunting of blood from the less vital organs of the shell to the vital core of the body. The "shell" is composed of the skin, digestive system, and skeletal musculature. The "core" includes the brain, heart, lungs, liver, and kidneys.

The shell/core effect accounts for the cool, pale skin observed in volume shock or cold response. It indicates that the body is trying to preserve the core at the expense of the shell. This can be a normal response to a minor, self-limiting problem, or the early sign of a more serious condition.

Swelling: Swelling is an increase in the pressure within body tissues due to the accumulation of excess fluid. This can come in the form of blood escaping from ruptured blood vessels (bleeding), or serum oozing from damaged capillaries

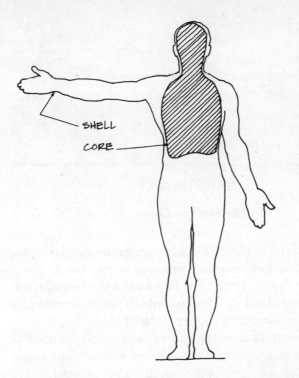

SHELL

CORE

(edema). It is a general response to injury or infection which occurs in all tissues. It may be localized, like the swelling of a sprained ankle, or systemic, like the swelling of the whole body that occurs in allergic reactions. Swelling can develop almost instantly, or slowly over the course of several hours.

Swelling which develops to the extent that it obstructs the flow of blood or air is the primary mechanism for most life-and-limb-threatening emergencies. It can be an immediate threat to life if the tissues affected are the vital organs of the BIG 3 (Circulatory, Respiratory, or Nervous Systems).

Anticipating or controlling the development of swelling is one of the keys to successful emergency care. Most of the swelling that occurs following injury develops during the first six hours. It then tapers off over the next eighteen hours, with very little swelling occurring after twenty-four hours. Re-injury can start the process over again.

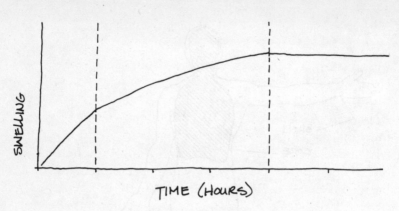

TIME (HOURS)

The Swelling Curve

Ischemia: This is the term for inadequate perfusion. Ischemia can occur when the perfusion pressure is too low to force blood into the tissues, or the pressure within the tissues is too high to allow the blood in. The most life-threatening examples of these problems occur in shock and head injury.

Ischemia can, of course, occur anywhere that perfusion is inadequate. If you were to wrap a string around your finger tight enough to reduce blood flow, the end of your finger would become "ischemic." If you left the string there long enough, the end of your finger would die.

Decompensation: In the presence of injury or illness, the Nervous System (brain) will make whatever changes are necessary in the functions of the Circulatory and Respiratory Systems to maintain perfusion and oxygenation. Early on, this compensation mechanism may work well enough to hide the problem. However, if the problem is serious, the normal compensatory responses will ultimately be overwhelmed. This is the condition known as decompensation.

Hopefully, however, by observing changes in vital signs in the context of other survey findings, we can detect compensation at work, and intervene to prevent decompensation. Recognizing the subtle changes of early compensation is another important key to saving lives in the backcountry.

For our purposes, the most sensitive and useful vital sign

is Level of Consciousness (C). This is due to the Nervous System's exquisite sensitivity to oxygen deprivation. Problems with perfusion and oxygenation are quickly indicated by changes in brain function.

Abnormal Consciousness: To understand nervous-system function as an indicator, picture the brain as a sort of onion with increasingly complex layers of function from the inside out. The basic "vegetative" functions of body regulation, breathing, and consciousness are contained in the deeper, more primitive layers. Higher functions such as personality, judgment, and problem solving would be located in the outer layers, added later in human evolution.

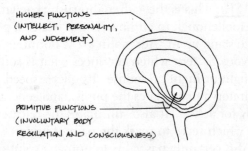

HIGHER FUNCTIONS
(INTELLECT, PERSONALITY, AND JUDGEMENT)

PRIMITIVE FUNCTIONS
(INVOLUNTARY BODY
REGULATION AND CONSCIOUSNESS)

The Evolutionary Onion

These outer layers, most recently acquired, are also the first to be lost when problems develop. The earliest vital sign changes seen are the beginning stages of "peeling the onion." We call this "Altered Mental Status." Patients remain conscious and alert, but may become anxious, uncooperative, or respond in ways that don't fit the situation. They may act intoxicated, belligerent, or confused.

More extreme injury effects the deeper layers, causing a decrease in level of consciousness. When the onion has peeled this far, the situation has become more serious. Patients progress from being alert (A) to lower levels of responsiveness (V,P), and unresponsiveness (U) as oxygen deprivation in brain tissue becomes more severe. The progression can also be reversed, if the underlying problems with perfusion and oxygenation are corrected.

Acute Stress Reaction (ASR): The acute stress reaction is a normal, self-limiting Nervous System response to acute stress of any type. The problem with ASR is that it can be mistaken for the symptoms of life-threatening conditions such as shock and increased intracranial pressure. For example, during ASR a shell/core effect actually occurs; the difference is that ASR is harmless and goes away with time. Acute Stress Reaction can also occur along with true shock, and cause problems by masking the symptoms of serious injury. ASR comes in two basic forms:

1. **Sympathetic (ASR):** This is the "adrenalin rush" known so well to those of us fool enough to climb over our heads or play in water too deep to stand up in. Adrenalin is the hormone released by the Nervous System which produces what is sometimes called the "fight or flight" response. Its effects speed up the pulse and respiratory rates, dilates the pupils, and generally gets the body ready for action. It also stimulates the release of natural hormones which serve to mask the pain of injury.

　　This type of ASR certainly has value to human evolution. It allows heroic survival efforts even in the presence of severe injury or other stress. However, it also makes the accurate assessment of injuries difficult for the rescuer in the time period immediately following the accident.

2. **Parasympathetic (ASR):** Feeling faint and nauseous in response to stress is another familiar feeling. It is caused by a temporary loss of perfusion to the brain due to a slowing of the heart rate. The evolutionary value of this response is more difficult to figure out. This, too, is harmless except in its ability to mimic the consciousness and mental status changes seen in shock and head injury. It is highly desirable to be able to distinguish ASR, which is self-limiting, from these serious conditions, especially in the backcountry.

3

BASIC LIFE SUPPORT

Discussing serious problems first has its drawbacks. You can get the feeling that every accident is going to produce some tragic and overwhelming injury. It can make you a bit shy about taking risks, or even letting yourself get more than a mile or two from a Level I trauma center. So keep in mind that we cover the big problems first because they're big, not because they're common.

GENERAL PRINCIPLES

REQUIREMENT FOR LIFE: Adequate perfusion of vital organs with oxygenated blood under all conditions.

LIFE-SAVING TREATMENT: *Perfuse the brain.* Any condition which has the potential to interfere with the flow of oxygen to the blood, or blood to the brain, must be corrected.

Basic Life Support (BLS) is the immediate treatment of life-threatening BIG 3 problems discovered during the Primary Survey. It should be your automatic response to conditions which are likely to cause death or severe disability. It is designed to provide temporary support for only the most vital functions of the Circulatory, Respiratory, and Nervous Systems while patient assessment continues, or until the patient is transferred to advanced treatment. For BLS to be effective, it must begin immediately at the scene.

Although BLS is outlined in a specific sequence, the reality of field treatment requires flexibility. In terms of saving lives, all BLS components are equally important. It is often necessary to change the order in which things are done, or to manage several components at the same time.

Most of the procedures used in Basic Life Support are covered by the Obstructed Airway and Cardiopulmonary Resuscitation (CPR) courses taught by the Red Cross and American Heart Association. We strongly recommend your participation in one of these courses. However, remember that it will require some flexibility to adapt what you learn there to the wilderness environment.

PRIMARY SURVEY

You'll remember from the chapter on the Patient Assessment System that the primary survey is a rapid look to see if the Circulatory, Respiratory and Nervous Systems are functioning. The simplest and most elegant way to conduct a primary survey is to ask your patient, "hey, how are you?" If she gives an appropriate verbal response such as "fine, will you help me get this rock off my foot?" you can be satisfied that there is no immediate life-threatening BIG 3 problem. Her airway is intact, she is breathing, her heart is beating, and her brain is functioning. You have done your primary survey. In cases where the patient is unable to respond, or has responded abnormally, you will need to look a little more closely. This is the process known as checking the ABCD's.

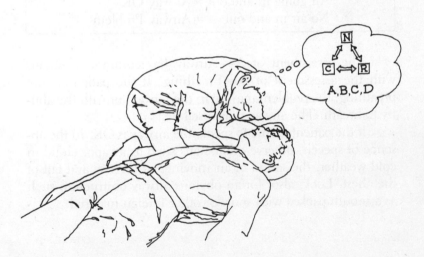

Primary Survey

A—AIRWAY

Airway problems in the Primary Survey are caused by obstruction of the Upper Airway (pharynx or larynx). Obstruction may be complete or partial. Complete obstruction is rapidly fatal, but can often be effectively treated with dramatic results. Possible causes of airway obstruction include: *Position:* Unconscious states produce relaxation of soft tissues ("swallowed his tongue"). *Vomit:* Most patients vomit at or near death. *Foreign Body:* Conscious people can inhale food. Children can inhale anything (coins, peanuts, etc.). Unconscious patients can also be obstructed by a foreign body (vomit, teeth, injured tissue). *Swelling:* Caused by trauma, irritants such as smoke or chemicals, or allergic reaction (anaphylaxis). *Spasm:* Sudden exposure to water can cause the throat to spasm. This accounts for infrequent cases of "dry drowning" where the lungs do not fill with water.

Primary Survey Assessment of A—Airway

Air going in and out = Airway OK
No air in and out   = Airway Problem

The assessment of A—Airway has common elements with the assessment of B—Breathing. If the patient is not breathing, the problem may be in the airway, or with the ability to breath. The airway is assessed first.

If the patient is able to speak, the airway is OK. In the absence of speech, observe other signs such as a vapor cloud in cold weather, the sound of air moving, or the rise and fall of the chest. Look, also, for an obvious airway obstruction such as a mouth packed with snow or other foreign material.

Primary Treatment of A—Airway Obstruction: Treatment of obstruction is a progression of actions from the most simple to the most desperate. Your hope is that the obstruction will be cleared without the need for significant movement of the patient.

The airway is opened using a jaw thrust, chin lift, or direct pull on the tongue while the neck is held in the in-line position to protect the spinal cord. Cervical spine stabilization is a component of BLS, so whenever there is the possibility of neck injury, positioning is done with minimal neck movement. Hyperextension of the neck, although taught in the past as an airway opening technique, adds little or nothing to the effect and can be extremely harmful if the spine is injured.

Try moving air into the patient's lungs with mouth-to-mouth breaths. If air does not go in, reposition the airway and try again. If air does goes in, the airway is not obstructed, the problem is B—Breathing.

If positioning and test breaths do not succeed in moving air, the cause of the obstruction is assumed to be foreign mate-

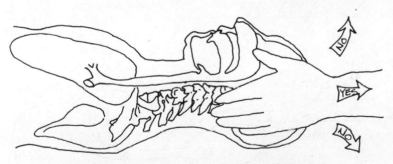

Gentle and steady "in-line" position protects the airway and the spinal cord.

rial. You must manually clear the airway. Try first to use gravity to clear obstructions. The usual method is to simply log-roll the whole patient to the side, keeping the spine in line, and "finger sweep" the mouth. If there is no mechanism for spine injury, roll the patient prone and pull up at the waist. This is effective in clearing vomit.

Another method is to use residual air to help clear obstructions. A sudden thrust to the abdomen or chest (the Heimlich maneuver) can force the air left in the patient's lungs out under pressure, blowing any obstruction out with it. The abdominal or chest thrust is done with the patient on his back. And, in cases where an obstructed patient is still conscious and standing, it is done from behind by grasping your own arms around the patient and squeezing. It really doesn't matter whether you are squeezing the abdomen or the chest, the effect is the same. For infants, the best method is to pound firmly on the patient's back between the shoulder blades while holding them head down.

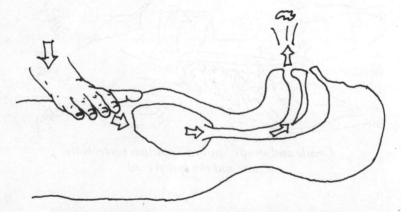

Abdominal or chest thrust—air trapped in the lungs can, under pressure, dislodge an obstruction.

B—BREATHING

Even with an open airway, the patient may not ventilate adequately. Inadequate ventilation means not enough air is moving in and out to support life. This can be the result of the lack of nervous system drive due to an injured spinal cord or the loss of brain function. It can also occur when the bellows mechanism of the chest wall and diaphragm is damaged.

Primary Assessment of B—Breathing:

```
Adequate ventilation    = Breathing OK
Inadequate ventilation  = Breathing not OK
```

"Not OK" and "Inadequate" are inexact terms. They generally refer to ventilation that is absent, very slow, or extremely irregular in an unconscious patient. Light-skinned individuals may turn pale or blue. If you are in doubt, consider the breathing inadequate and begin to support ventilation. In the conscious patient, ask for a verbal response. A person who is able to speak generally has ventilation adequate for the Primary Survey.

Primary Treatment of B—Breathing: Inadequate or absent ventilation is treated by blowing into the lungs through the airway. This is called positive pressure ventilation (PPV) or artificial respiration (AR). The rate of ventilation should be about 12 breaths per minute (one every 5 seconds) or faster. Volume is adequate when you can see the chest rise slightly. Each breath is done slowly over 1–1½ seconds. Faster flow rates tend to blow air into the stomach, leading to gastric distension and vomiting.

Patients who are breathing on their own, but not deeply or frequently enough, can be assisted with ventilation timed to blow air in with the patient's own inspiratory effort. This is especially useful in treating inadequate respiration due to chest wall injury.

C—CIRCULATION—Pulse

Cardiac arrest refers to the loss of effective heart activity. No pulse can be felt. Cardiac arrest immediately leads to loss of consciousness and respiratory arrest due to loss of brain perfusion. A *patient who is at all responsive (A, V, P on the AVPU scale), breathing, or moving spontaneously is NOT in cardiac arrest.*

Primary Assessment of Pulse

Pulse   = Circulation OK
No pulse = Circulation not OK

Pulses can be very difficult to find under adverse field conditions such as fear, cold hands, dangerous places, and so on. The pulse is very weak in the presence of shock, and very slow if the patient is in profound hypothermia. It is extremely important to take the time to find a pulse. The carotid pulse is the easiest to get to, and the strongest to feel. It is located on either side of the adam's apple (larynx) in the neck. If the carotid pulse is absent, the heart is not beating.

➡ *Treatment of Pulselessness—CPR:* Cardiopulmonary Resuscitation (CPR) is a combination of chest compressions and ventilation (PPV) which produces some perfusion of the brain and vital organs. The generally accepted procedures for chest compressions and ventilation are outlined in the American Heart Association guidelines for CPR.

CPR has limited application in the backcountry. The patient's own natural heart activity must be restored within a short period of time if the patient is to survive. This usually requires Advanced Life Support (ALS) with drugs and electrical defibrillation.

Although ventilation can support breathing for hours or days, chest compressions cannot support circulation for a prolonged period of time. Most medical authorities agree that the chances of survival are minimal if spontaneous heart activity is not restored within about 30 minutes. The exceptions to this are in cases of severe hypothermia, and in cold-water drowning.

Chest compressions cannot preserve life in situations where the cardiac arrest occurs as a result of massive trauma to the chest, severe blood loss, spinal cord transection, or massive head injury. In these cases it is best to realize that the patient has died. It is not necessary or useful to start or continue CPR when these conditions are discovered.

C—CIRCULATION—Bleeding

Adequate perfusion requires sufficient circulating blood volume. Blood loss must be controlled as part of the BLS process. Bleeding can be external and obvious, or internal and more difficult to detect and stop.

Primary Assessment of Severe Bleeding: External bleeding is usually obvious, but can be missed when a full exam is not done. Snow can make bleeding less obvious because blood tends to quickly melt through and disappear. Bulky clothing can absorb or obscure blood with the same effect.

Bleeding from an artery is usually the most immediately life threatening. It will be under pressure and may spurt with the pulsing of the heart. There is no easy rule for deciding when bleeding is severe. Generally, if it looks like a lot of blood, it probably is.

Internal bleeding is not so obvious and will generally not be discovered in the Primary Survey. It can usually be inferred by a history of trauma with the development of shock. Severe internal bleeding is frequently associated with fractures of the femur and pelvis, and blunt abdominal and chest injury.

➡ ***Primary Treatment of Severe Bleeding:*** All bleeding stops eventually, we'd just like to do it while the patient still has enough blood to appreciate our efforts. External bleeding is controlled by well aimed direct pressure over the bleeding site. Pressure can be applied with the bare hand if necessary, but a bandage or cloth is preferred if available. This is not to absorb blood, but to provide even pressure across the damaged vessels.

If bleeding continues, remove the bandage and look again for the source of blood, and re-aim your pressure. You should expect to apply pressure for 10 or more minutes before a clot will form. Once bleeding is controlled, a pressure bandage should be applied. Beware, however, of obstructing circulation by creating an accidental tourniquet. Tourniquets are used only for major amputations if direct pressure is not effective.

D—DISABILITY—*Spine*

Injuries to the vertebrae of the spine can damage the spinal cord with dramatic, devastating, and permanent results. It

Well-aimed direct pressure stops severe bleeding.

is essential that management of spine injury be considered part of Basic Life Support. The most dangerous movement of the cervical spine is flexion (movement of the chin toward the chest). Moderate extension is usually safe. Hyperextension (tilting the head back) is dangerous. (Refer to the illustration on p. 55, "In-Line Position" (neck).)

Primary Assessment of Spine Injury: Any event that could possibly produce spine injury is a positive mechanism. This is one of the factors you determine in your survey of the scene. Examples include a fall from a cliff, being tumbled by an avalanche, or a long swim over a short waterfall. No further exam is necessary, these are all treated as spine injuries *during the Primary Survey.* The spine itself will be examined during the Secondary Survey and the possibility of injury can then be reevaluated.

Primary Treatment of Spine Injury: If no movement of the spine is required for treatment, or is likely to occur during your exam, leave things as they are while you complete your Patient Assessment. If you must move the spine, do so while applying Traction Into Position (TIP—see page 117.) This brings the head and neck into the neutral (eyes forward) position. Continue manual TIP during Basic Life Support and the rest of the patient assessment. Spine splints are applied after the PAS is finished.

The airway can be managed effectively and safely with the neck held by traction in position. If it is necessary to roll the patient to clear vomit, hold the head, neck, and trunk in line as a unit (log roll).

D—DISABILITY—*Consciousness*

Abnormal consciousness indicates Nervous System problems severe enough to affect the brain. Because it is an indicator of BIG 3 function, consciousness is included in the Primary Survey.

Primary Assessment of Consciousness: AVPU (see page 37) is a relatively precise and universally understood scale. It replaces subjective terms such as "semi-conscious" that are often vague and confusing.

➡ **Primary Treatment Level of Consciousness Changes:** There is no specific treatment in Basic Life Support for the Nervous System problems indicated by AVPU changes. Treatment is aimed at the life-threatening Airway / Breathing / Circulation problems which are causing the Nervous System changes.

SECTION II

THE
BIG 3
BODY
SYSTEMS

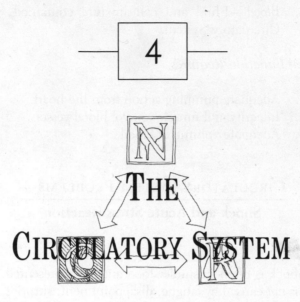

4

THE CIRCULATORY SYSTEM

STRUCTURE AND FUNCTION

To effectively perfuse the body tissues with oxygenated blood, the Circulatory System requires adequate pumping action from the heart and integrity of the vessels to maintain perfusion pressure. It also requires an adequate volume of blood. To complete its part in the BIG 3 triad, the Circulatory System must have oxygen faithfully supplied to the lungs by the Respiratory System, and good Nervous System control of heart rate and blood-vessel pressure.

Three Major Components

1. *Heart*—Maintains blood flow and pressure through pumping action.
2. *Blood Vessels*—Contain blood volume. Able to help maintain pressure through constriction controlled by Nervous System.

3. *Blood*—Fluid and cell mixture contained within Circulatory System.

Normal Function Requires

1. Adequate pumping action from the heart.
2. Integrity and muscle tone of blood vessels.
3. Adequate volume of blood.

CIRCULATORY SYSTEM PROBLEMS—
Shock and Acute Stress Reaction

SHOCK

Shock is often misunderstood and misrepresented. True shock is *not* caused by fatigue, disappointment, surprise, grief, or any other reaction to *psychological* stress. These factors often cause a condition called "Acute Stress Reaction" which can look like shock, but has none of the serious consequences. True shock is a *physiologic* condition caused by an acute loss of perfusion pressure in the Circulatory System. Shock can be the result of failure of the pumping action of the heart, dilation or leaking of the blood vessels, or loss of blood volume. True shock always indicates a life-threatening physical condition which requires specific, aggressive treatment, preferably in the hospital. It does not spontaneously improve in the field. Without treatment, the patient will die.

The classic symptoms of shock are pale skin, elevated heart rate, and elevated respiratory rate, all caused by the body's attempt to compensate for loss of normal perfusion pressure. Shock develops along a spectrum of severity from mild to severe. Progression can be stopped at any given point, but it is more common for shock to progress from bad to worse. There are various types of shock, but the most commonly encountered in backcountry emergencies is volume shock.

In trauma, sudden loss of circulating blood volume is usually the result of internal or external bleeding. However, blood volume can also be lost indirectly over hours or days through dehydration. The fluid one loses as sweat, vomit, or diarrhea will ultimately result in reduced fluid volume in the blood stream.

Assessment of Shock: A history of trauma sufficient to cause severe internal or external bleeding should make you think immediately of volume shock. This is also true of severe fluid loss from diarrhea, vomiting or sweating. The classic sign of cool and pale skin is caused by the shell/core effect during compensation. This particular sign may be less than useful in cold environments as the shell/core effect is also part of the body's normal protection against heat loss.

The vital sign pattern shows the compensation mechanisms at work. A loss of blood volume or other body fluid results in an emergency effort to maintain perfusion to vital organs. The degree of change in vital signs reflects the severity of the fluid loss.

The first vital sign change to occur as shock develops is an increase in heart rate, followed closely by an increase in the respiratory rate. If you are able to measure blood pressure, you will observe that it remains near normal early on, which shows that the compensatory mechanisms are working. In long-term care, urine output is a good measurement of available fluid in the core circulation. Reduced blood volume will be reflected in greatly reduced urine output.

In the early stages of shock, this compensation mechanism may work so well that it prevents symptoms from being noticed. As long as the brain remains adequately perfused, the patient's mental functions will be fairly normal. However, as the shell/core compensation mechanism is overwhelmed (decompensation), perfusion to the brain is reduced and the "onion" starts to peel. The higher brain functions (personality, problem-solving ability, etc.) are the most sensitive to decreased perfusion. As shock progresses, compensation will fail, perfusion pressure will fall, and level of consciousness will decay.

VITAL SIGNS IN VOLUME SHOCK

	NORMAL	MILD	MODERATE	SEVERE
BP:	>110/64	normal	decreased	decreased
P:	72	<100	100–120	>120
R:	12	14–20	20–35	>35
C:	Alert	anxious	anxious	V, P or U
T:	98.6	normal	normal	normal
S:	Normal	normal or pale	pale cool	pale cool
Urine Output:	>30 ml/ hour	decreased	decreased	none

➡ *Treatment of Shock:* Shock is generally a serious BIG 3 problem that you cannot treat effectively in the backcountry. The traditional "treatments" of reassurance, elevating the feet, and keeping warm are certainly good for any patient in shock, but does nothing to address the real problem of low blood volume. A patient in shock needs intravenous (IV) fluids, surgeons, and a hospital. This is a bona fide emergency and you are justified in recruiting whatever help is necessary to get the patient to advanced medical care. The only real field treatment for shock is evacuation. There are, of course, temporary measures which may help stabilize the situation long enough to reach medical care.

ACUTE STRESS REACTION (ASR)

Following sudden stress or injury which may or may not be serious, a variety of reactions including extreme anxiety, feeling dazed or disoriented, fainting, hyperventilating, and pain masking sometimes called "psychogenic shock" or Acute

GENERIC TEMPORARY
TREATMENT FOR SHOCK

Stop Volume Loss: Maintaining full volume is helpful for any type of shock. In the field, this usually means the control of external bleeding. Internal bleeding and other types of fluid loss may be impossible to control in the wilderness setting.

All external bleeding can be stopped by well aimed direct pressure, with or without bandages. If direct pressure on the bleeding site does not seem to be working, you are either not applying enough pressure or you are in the wrong place. Take your hand and the bandage away, look for the source of the blood, and try again. Pressure points and tourniquets (except in cases of complete amputation) are much less effective.

Position: Lying flat with legs elevated works with gravity to perfuse core organs. This is the textbook "treatment" for shock found in every first-aid book. This position may be helpful, but it is certainly not definitive treatment. Warmth and reassurance are also helpful, but not definitive either. Protection from heat loss is important for *any* patient exposed to the environment and unable to exercise to maintain body heat.

Fluids: Sometimes brought to the scene by rescue teams, intravenous fluids infused rapidly and directly into the circulatory system can help restore volume. This is only a temporary measure to stabilize the patient during evacuation.

In cases where mild shock is developing slowly due to sweating or diarrhea, drinking fluids may reverse the problem. However, this is a very slow method of fluid replacement which will not be very effective if shock is more severe, or fluid loss is rapid.

Oxygen: Supplemental oxygen may be brought to the scene by rescue teams if weight and time constraints allow. Supplemental oxygen is also only a temporary measure, and has limited effect in the field setting.

Stress Reaction (ASR) commonly occur (See Section I, Chapter 2). Because these reactions are also under the control of the Nervous System they may appear similar to true shock or the compensation mechanism of volume shock.

The use of the term psychogenic "shock" for this phenomenon can be confusing and misleading because the consequences are very different from true shock. It is important to distinguish true shock, in its various degrees of compensation and levels of severity, from an acute stress reaction which might look similar but is not at all life-threatening.

In the hospital or ambulance setting the difference is less important since both are managed as shock. For long-term management in the wilderness, however, recognizing ASR for what it is, when possible, can save a lot of emergency resources, not to mention your peace of mind.

Assessment of ASR: The key to recognizing Acute Stress Reaction is in the mechanism of injury and the progression of symptoms. ASR can look like shock, but can occur with or without any mechanism of injury which can cause shock. Also, with the passage of time, ASR will get better, especially with calm reassurance.

We have all seen people with only minor extremity sprains or superficial wounds become lightheaded, pale, and nauseated. Although they look "shocky," there is no cause for alarm, and certainly no need for helicopters and emergency surgery. They have no mechanism for sudden volume loss. We let them lay down and they get better.

It is important to remember that Acute Stress Reaction can co-exist with true shock. In cases where the patient has both a good reason to be in true shock, and the signs and symptoms to go with it, you must treat it as such.

Field Treatment of ASR: Allowing the patient to lie down, providing calm reassurance, and relieving pain by treating injuries should result in immediate improvement in symptoms. Note that this is the traditional "treatment for shock" described in many first aid texts.

CASE STUDY

S: An 18-year-old man skiing out-of-bounds fell against a stump injuring his left upper leg. He was unable to move without extreme pain, and was forced to lie in the snow until he was discovered about an hour later. The skier who found him was also alone, and immediately left the scene to report a "dead body" on the slope. By that time it was just past sunset. The air temperature was −5 degrees with a moderate north wind.

O: Ski patrollers found the patient lying on his back in the snow. Ski tracks in the powder exposed a large spruce stump. The patient's airway was clear and he was breathing. The only response noted was a weak grimace when the patroller doing his Secondary Survey touched the patient's left thigh. Even through ski clothing, the patroller could feel that the leg was quite swollen. Vital Signs at 17:40—BP: unknown, P: 120, R: 24, C: P on AVPU scale, Skin: pale, T: feels cold.

A: 1. Volume Shock
2. Fracture L Femur
3. Unreliable Exam, can't rule out spine injury

A': Severe Hypothermia

P: The patient was placed in cervical immobilization using a blanket roll. The limbs were aligned using Traction Into Position, and the patient was wrapped in blankets and a plastic tarp and immobilized in the toboggan. During the ride down the mountain, the patrollers stopped every minute to check airway and breathing. They arrived at the First-Aid Station twenty minutes later. The patient was transferred immediately to an ambulance for the one-hour ride to the hospital.

Discussion: This fellow arrived at the hospital, alive, with a body core temperature of 94.4, in compensated volume shock. His left femur was fractured and the femoral artery lacerated.

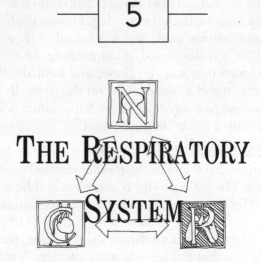

THE RESPIRATORY SYSTEM

STRUCTURE AND FUNCTION

One of the BIG 3 body systems, the Respiratory System performs the task of bringing adequate quantities of outside air into close proximity to blood (Circulatory System). This takes place in the alveoli of the lungs where only a thin membrane separates air from blood, allowing the diffusion of oxygen into the blood, and carbon dioxide out of the blood.

The rest of the system consists of semi-rigid tubes to conduct air to the alveoli, and a bellows system for moving the air in and out. Like the Circulatory System, the Respiratory System is under Nervous System control. Under normal conditions, the brain measures the pH (acidity) of the blood which is a reflection of the amount of carbon dioxide (CO_2) dissolved in it. Too much CO_2 in the blood causes the pH to drop. The brain responds by increasing the rate and depth of respiration to "blow off" the CO_2 until a normal pH is reestablished. Conversely, too little CO_2 is corrected by decreasing the rate and depth of respiration.

The Respiratory System contains five major components:

1.   *Upper Airway*—Consists of the mouth (Oropharynx), nose (Nasopharynx), and throat (Larynx).
2.   *Lower Airway*—Composed of large tubes (Trachea), smaller tubes (Bronchi), and the smallest tubes (Bronchioles).
3.   *Alveoli*—The terminal membranous air sacks at the end of the system, adjacent to blood-filled capillaries where oxygen and carbon dioxide exchange occurs.

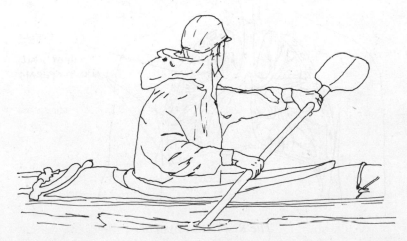

4. *Chest Wall/Diaphragm*—In normal function, similar to a bellows. Inspiration (the intake of air) is caused by the active contraction of the diaphragm and chest-wall muscles, which expand the rib cage sucking air into the lungs. Expiration (air out) is a passive process which occurs when these muscles relax and the natural elasticity of the lungs and chest squeeze the air out.

5. *Nervous System Drive*—The Nervous System (brain) controls the rate and depth of respiration in response to the amount of carbon dioxide and oxygen in the blood.

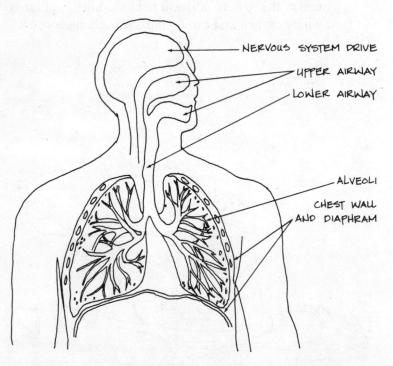

The Respiratory System

Normal function of the Respiratory System requires:

1. Clear upper airway
2. Clear lower airway
3. Alveoli with membrane exposed to air
4. Functioning bellows
5. Intact Nervous System

RESPIRATORY SYSTEM PROBLEMS

There are dozens of different Respiratory System problems which can develop directly, or be the indirect result of Circulatory or Nervous System problems. They all have the same effect; reduced oxygen supply to the blood (except hyperventilation syndrome). We can condense these problems into five broad categories, which are given the same generic treatment, with a few additional specifics. Since the generic treatment applies to all respiratory problems, we'll outline it first.

UPPER AIRWAY OBSTRUCTION

The upper airway may be obstructed by the tongue, a piece of food, or the fact that the patient's head is under water. Obstruction can also be the result of swelling from trauma or infection.

Assessment of Airway Obstruction: If the primary survey reveals the absence of respiration, even if the patient is still conscious, Basic Life Support procedures are instituted immediately (see Chapter 3, page 54).

If airway obstruction is not complete, the patient may have noisy and difficult respiration. The ability to swallow is often impaired, and the patient may be drooling. Talking may be difficult or impossible.

GENERIC TREATMENT FOR RESPIRATORY DISTRESS

Position—Any patient in respiratory distress, who is able to move, will already have found the best position in which to breathe. This is usually sitting up to allow gravity to assist the diaphragm, and to help keep fluids out of the airway tubes. In unconscious or immobile patients, special care must be taken to position them in a way that prevents airway obstruction from secretions, vomit, or the collapse of their own airway (see BLS section, p. 54). This is usually on the patient's side, with the head and neck in the "in line" position.

Reassurance—Encourage the patient to breathe slower and deeper, rather than panting like a dog. This brings in fresh oxygen rather than moving the same old carbon dioxide back and forth in the tubes.

Ventilation—A patient in respiratory distress will fatigue rapidly. You may need to provide assistance with "positive pressure ventilation," timed to coincide with the patient's own efforts. This positive-pressure ventilation is produced by the rescuer blowing air in as the patient tries to inhale and can often work when the patient cannot draw in air on his or her own.

Oxygen—If available, giving supplemental oxygen will increase the concentration of oxygen getting into the blood, and ultimately, to the brain.

Assessment of partial obstruction is directed at determining if the patient is getting enough air to support life until medical care can be reached. You are looking for signs that oxygenation of the blood is adequate; good skin color, minimal changes in consciousness and mental status (A on the AVPU scale), and no worsening of the respiratory distress.

Treatment of Airway Obstruction: For the treatment of complete airway obstruction, or partial obstruction with inadequate oxygenation, refer to Basic Life Support (Chapter 3).

In cases where a foreign object is lodged in the throat for a brief time and successfully removed before the patient gets in real trouble, you may certainly congratulate yourself on a real "save." However, be aware that the object may have caused sufficient irritation to result in later swelling, which is another form of obstruction. Such a patient should be closely watched, and an evacuation begun if necessary.

In cases of partial airway obstruction with adequate oxygenation, the rule is "do no harm." Apply the generic treatment for respiratory distress and evacuate quickly. In almost all cases of partial obstruction, breathing cool air will reduce swelling of the airway temporarily. Be prepared to perform airway opening maneuvers detailed in Basic Life Support if it becomes apparent that the airway is closing. A partial obstruction frequently becomes worse over time.

LOWER AIRWAY CONSTRICTION

Spasm, swelling, or the accumulation of mucus or pus can cause narrowing of the lower airway tubes (bronchi and bronchioles). This is what happens in asthma, bronchitis, and anaphylaxis. The effect is to slow the movement of air in and out of the lung tissue.

Assessment of Lower Airway Constriction: Expiration is often prolonged, with wheezing and gurgling. Sometimes, the lower airway noise is loud enough to hear from a distance. Other times you may need a stethoscope or an ear to the patient's chest.

The patient may recall exposure to smoke, inhaled water, or other irritating substances indicating a generalized swelling. He may have been exposed to something to which he is allergic, indicating anaphylaxis. Or, there may be a history of slowly worsening illness and fever, pointing to respiratory infection. Whatever the cause, the patient usually develops a cough as the Respiratory System tries to clear itself. There may be an obvious increase in respiratory effort as the system struggles to move air against increased resistance.

Vital signs may show increases in the compensatory mechanisms with elevated heart and respiratory rates. The presence of fever may indicate a respiratory infection.

➤ Treatment of Lower Airway Constriction:
1. Generic Treatment for Respiratory Distress (see page 76)
2. Specific Treatment for Lower Airway Constriction: Treatment with antibiotics for infection, and/or bronchodilators for asthma may be necessary. In the presence of respiratory distress, evacuation is indicated.

PULMONARY FLUID

Excess fluid accumulates in air sacs (alveoli) blocking the exchange of oxygen and carbon dioxide between air and blood. This may come from outside the system, or from within. The most common sources are: *Aspiration*—Vomit or other foreign material is inhaled. *Drowning*—Water is inhaled in "wet drowning." *Pulmonary Edema*—Fluid may leak from Circulatory System capillaries into the alveoli (air sacs). This can be the result of too much pressure in the capillaries from congestive heart failure, swelling in reaction to irritants like water and smoke, or the effects of high altitude. *Bleeding*—Contusion or laceration of the lung tissue may cause alveoli to fill with blood. *Pneumonia*—Infection fills the air sacs with pus.

Assessment of Pulmonary Fluid: Large amounts of fluid in the lungs will cause gurgling which can be heard at a distance. Fluid may actually froth at the mouth ("talking in bubbles").

Small amounts of fluid may be heard with an ear to the chest as "crackling" on respiration. Vital signs will show that the body is compensating for partial loss of lung function with an increase in respiratory and heart rates. The development of fever indicates infection.

In less severe cases, this loss of lung function may not be noticed while the patient is at rest. However, with the increased demands of exercise, the reduced lung capacity will become obvious as the patient becomes short of breath much more easily than normal.

Coughing is common with the accumulation of pulmonary fluid. It may produce sputum tinged with pus or blood. There may be a history of injury to lung tissue through exposure to smoke, infection, or near drowning. Or, you may have just arrived at 12,000 feet on your ascent of Mt. Logan and be experiencing the beginning of high-altitude pulmonary edema.

Treatment of Pulmonary Fluid:
1. Generic Treatment for Respiratory Distress (see page 76)
2. Specific Treatment for Pulmonary Fluid: Evacuation to medical care. In high-altitude sickness, immediate descent to a lower altitude.

CHEST TRAUMA

Trauma to the chest wall or airway tubes can interfere with the function of the Respiratory System in a number of ways. The injuries are usually complicated and severe, and cannot be effectively managed in the field. Chest trauma with respiratory distress is best evacuated without delay.

Lung contusion is the term applied to the development of generic swelling in the lung tissue following injury. The chest wall remains stable with the bellows system intact, but pulmonary fluid begins to accumulate in the alveoli. This can occur along with suspected rib fracture, or any severe blow to the chest.

An unstable chest wall, also called a "flail chest," indicates that the bellows system is damaged to the point that it is no longer rigid. The chest wall collapses with inspiration causing incomplete lung expansion.

Hemothorax and pneumothorax are terms used to describe the presence of blood (heme), or air (pneumo) in the chest cavity (thorax). This blood and/or air occupies the space between the lungs and the chest wall, preventing full expansion of the lungs even though the bellows may continue to operate. In the case of an open pneumothorax, sometimes called a "sucking chest wound," air may enter the chest cavity through an injury in the chest wall. In a closed pneumothorax, air may enter the chest cavity through an injured lung. It may affect only one side or both.

Assessment of Chest Trauma: There will be a history of significant blunt trauma to the chest, or evidence of penetrating injury. There may be bruising, fractured ribs, or other evidence of potential injury to lungs or chest wall. In the presence of chest-wall injury or hemopneumothorax there may be a radical decrease in respiratory function, even though the patient is obviously making a great effort to breathe. It will be apparent by level of consciousness and mental-status changes, and other vital signs, that the patient is not getting enough oxygen. Significant injury to the Circulatory System also often occurs with severe chest trauma, and will result in volume shock.

Treatment of Chest Trauma:

1. Generic Treatment for Respiratory Distress (see page 76).
Like the "treatment for shock," this is limited and temporary
only. The patient with chest injury significant enough to cause
respiratory distress requires immediate evacuation.

2. Specific Treatment for Chest Trauma: Lying on the injured side reduces pain and may reduce instability. Gravity
can help keep blood from building up in the uninjured side of
the chest. In case of a simple rib fracture, a wide bandage
wrapped around the chest can make the patient more comfortable and thus better able to control breathing.

In cases of open chest wounds, the injury should be covered with an air-tight seal, like a piece of plastic bag. This will
stop the "sucking" chest wound from allowing air into the
chest cavity instead of the lungs. If the patch works the way it
should, respiration and oxygenation should improve. If symptoms become worse, the patch should be removed.

DECREASED NERVOUS-SYSTEM DRIVE

Breathing is controlled by the Nervous System. If the
Nervous System ceases to function, breathing will stop (respiratory arrest). The causes include toxins and drugs, head injury, altitude sickness, lightning strike, and hypothermia.

Assessment of Decreased Nervous-System Drive: As respiratory drive decreases for whatever reason, respiratory rate and
depth decreases, becomes irregular, or stops. The difference
between adequate and inadequate respiration is not always
clear. Vital signs are likely to be affected by whatever the Nervous System problem is, and therefore are not reliable indicators of whether or not the patient is getting enough oxygen.
However, anyone with pale or blue skin, slowed or irregular
breathing, and reduced level of consciousness should be considered to be in need of treatment for respiratory distress.

➡ *Treatment for Decreased Nervous-System Drive:*
1. Basic Life Support (Chapter 3).
2. Generic Treatment for Respiratory Distress (page 76)
3. Evacuation: Correcting the Nervous System problem is not something you're likely to do in the field.

HYPERVENTILATION (INCREASED NERVOUS-SYSTEM DRIVE)

Increased respiratory drive normally occurs with altitude, exercise, and other physiological demands. Abnormal increase in respiration occurs with Acute Stress Reaction (See Chapter 4, page 68). The result can be an abnormal decrease in the carbon-dioxide concentration in the blood with the pH increasing. This is blood chemistry out of balance, which can effect the Nervous System. This is usually referred to as "hyperventilation syndrome."

Assessment of Hyperventilation: Hyperventilation can occur with or without obvious fast and heavy breathing. It only takes a slight increase in depth and rate over time to cause changes in blood pH. The respiratory changes observed in your measurement of vital signs may be very subtle.

It can be difficult to distinguish between hyperventilation syndrome and serious Respiratory or Nervous System problems, especially if there is a positive mechanism for injury. As with other components of Acute Stress Reaction, however, it gets significantly better with time and basic treatment.

There are some classic Nervous System effects of hyperventilation worth mentioning. Tingling of hands and feet occurs with most moderate and severe reactions. Tingling and numbness around the mouth is also common. The ability to move extremities voluntarily is unaffected.

Treatment of Hyperventilation:
1. Generic Treatment for Respiratory Distress (p. 76)
2. Specific Treatment for Hyperventilation Syndrome: Reassurance is specific and effective. Patients generally feel better with an explanation of their symptoms and can be "coached" to breath slower. When you are certain that hyperventilation is the only problem, breathing into a paper bag is occasionally used to artificially increase the concentration of CO_2 in the air inhaled. This seems to work, probably mostly by placebo effect.

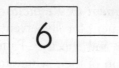

6

THE NERVOUS SYSTEM

STRUCTURE AND FUNCTION

The Nervous System consists of the brain, spinal cord, and peripheral nerves. The brain, in addition to being responsible for remembering where you left your flashlight, controls all critical life functions. Its primary connection with the Circulatory and Respiratory Systems is through the spinal cord. Both the brain and cord are encased within the bony structure of the skull and vertebrae of the spine.

From the gaps between vertebrae, peripheral nerves branch out from the spinal cord to all body tissues. Nerves controlling the most critical functions exit the cord at the base of the skull, and in the neck. This is why spinal cord injuries that occur in this area can cause extreme disability or death due to the loss of Nervous System control over vital body functions.

All Nervous System tissue is extremely sensitive to injury, especially oxygen deprivation. The most highly evolved functions of the brain, such as intellect and personality, are the most susceptible. For example, reduced perfusion due to shock will affect mental status before it affects the more primitive respiratory drive centers of the brain. This is why changes in mental status are often the best first indicators of a developing life-threatening condition.

The Nervous System consists of two major components:

1. *The Central Nervous System*—Consists of the brain and spinal cord encased in the bony protection of the skull and spine.
2. *The Peripheral Nervous System*—Composed of the unprotected nerves running between the central nervous system and the body tissues. These nerves typically run in bundles along with arteries and veins.

Normal Nervous-System function requires:

1. Uninterrupted perfusion of the Central Nervous System with oxygenated blood.
2. Intact central and peripheral nerve pathways between the Central Nervous System and the body tissues.

NERVOUS SYSTEM PROBLEMS

INCREASED INTRACRANIAL PRESSURE (ICP)

The brain, like other body tissues, will swell from bleeding and edema when injured. Unlike other tissues, however, the brain is confined within the rigid structure of the skull (cranium) where there simply is not much additional space to accommodate swelling. Therefore, injury to the brain, or other intracranial tissues, can produce a dangerous rise in intracranial pressure which can prevent adequate perfusion with oxygenated blood. Common causes include severe head injury, stroke, and high-altitude cerebral edema (HACE).

Assessment of Increased ICP: Like shock, increased ICP has a typical pattern and spectrum of severity, regardless of its cause or rate of onset.

History—Look for a mechanism for injury to brain tissue such as trauma, suffocation, or altitude.

Abnormal Consciousness—Although other vital-sign changes occur, alteration of consciousness and mental status is the most sensitive early indicator of increased ICP. This is the peeling of the "evolutionary onion" again. The patient may appear "drunk," or become combative or restless early, with decrease on the AVPU scale as ICP progresses. *It can be very difficult or impossible to tell the difference between a patient who is intoxicated by alcohol or drugs, and someone with increased ICP.*

Vomiting—Persistent vomiting is also a relatively reliable early indicator of problems with ICP.

Headache—Severe headache is an early sign of increased ICP. However, it is easily confused with pain from an injured neck, scalp, or skull.

Unequal Pupils—This sign is worthy of special mention because it is frequently cited as evidence of brain injury, even in patients showing no mental-status changes. However, this is a late sign in ICP. It occurs only with or after significant changes in consciousness. An alert, oriented person with unequal pupils either has an eye problem, or is just built that way. Don't rely on this sign out of context.

Other Signs—Paralysis, seizures, irregular breathing, or other signs of BIG 3 problems may also develop late in the progress of ICP. They may follow consciousness and mental status changes by minutes, hours, or days.

Treatment of Increased ICP: Unfortunately, field treatment will have little effect on the patient's chances for recovery. Surgery is generally required to relieve pressure and stop intracranial bleeding. The rapid onset of severe swelling from intracranial bleeding will probably be fatal in most backcountry settings.

However, early recognition of swelling which may be developing more slowly can save lives. As long as the patient remains alive, there are steps you can take to give the injured person a chance. The key is good basic life support and rapid evacuation with special attention to protection of the cervical spine and the airway. As long as there is a heart beat, there is a chance of at least partial recovery from severe head injury. Once the heart has stopped, however, there is little or no chance for recovery.

CONCUSSION (MINOR HEAD INJURY)

"Head injury" is an often misused term. It refers specifically to an injury *to the brain*. It is important to distinguish head injury with its Nervous-System signs, from injuries to the scalp or face which do not involve brain injury. These are referred to as "head wounds."

Minor head injury, usually referred to as "concussion," occurs when the patient strikes his head while falling, or something falls on the patient's head. The event results in a temporary loss of some neurological function, indicating that the brain has suffered some degree of injury, although ICP is not elevated.

Assessment of Minor Head Injury: Typically, the patient experiences a brief loss of consciousness (V or P on the AVPU scale) or lapse of memory. There may be a short period of disorientation or loss of memory for the event itself ("what happened, how did I get here?"). He may feel dazed, sleepy, or nauseated.

Assessment is directed at determining whether the injured brain tissue will swell enough in the next twenty-four hours to increase ICP. Will this minor concussion become a severe head injury?

This is one of the classic backcountry medical dilemmas; to evacuate now, or wait and watch.

There are no absolute rules, but there some general guidelines. Minor head injuries associated with RED FLAGS are more likely to become serious problems.

RED FLAGS
FOR MINOR HEAD INJURY

—Any decline in consciousness or mental status following an injury.
—The patient vomits or complains of severe headache.

Treatment of Minor Head Injury: Concussion requires no specific field treatment. However, it is important to monitor the patient carefully for at least twenty-four hours to detect the onset of increased ICP. Patients being monitored should not use narcotic or stimulant drugs, or drink alcohol. These would make the assessment of consciousness and mental-status changes very difficult.

Generally, in a remote backcountry setting, it is best to begin the evacuation of patients with confirmed concussion, rather than wait for the onset of ICP. This is especially true of patients with RED FLAG signs and symptoms. We also must remember to evaluate and treat for C-spine (cervical-spine) injury, which has the same mechanism of injury.

In less remote settings, you might choose to camp closer to a road for a day. If you're on the water, you might want to alter course to sail closer inshore as you monitor your patient over the next twenty-four hours.

SEIZURES

Brain tissue has electrical properties much like heart tissue. Seizures are caused by an uncoordinated burst of electrical activity in the brain. They have a variety of causes.

Assessment of Seizures: The important consideration in assessment is the context in which the seizure occurs. Seizures can be part of the pattern of increased ICP in trauma patients, or a relatively expected occurrence in a patient with epilepsy. They can be related to drug use, or occur for no apparent reason in an otherwise healthy individual.

The classic "grand mal" seizure is characterized by generalized tensing of all body muscles and repetitive, purposeless movement. Although the eyes may be open, the patient will be unresponsive during the seizure. He may be incontinent of feces and urine. There will usually be a period of drowsiness and disorientation after the seizure has ended.

Treatment of Seizure: Protection from injury is the most important treatment that you can provide the patient during the seizure. Most will resolve spontaneously in a short period of time. Protect the patient from injury when falling or thrashing. Common layman's "treatment," like chest compressions and trying to force objects between the teeth, are unnecessary and should be avoided.

Seizing patients will normally hold their breath for a short period of time and become cyanotic (blue). This is not a problem as long as it does not last more than a couple of minutes. Position the patient and ventilate if necessary after the seizure has resolved. Be prepared to open and clear the airway, if necessary, once the seizure has ended.

The real worry, of course, is not the seizure itself but what has caused it. Unless the patient is a known epileptic who has frequent seizures, the cause must be researched by a neurologist. Since the seizure may be the first sign of a serious condition, evacuation is a good idea.

SPINAL CORD—TRAUMA

The delicate tissue of the spinal cord, really an extension of the brain, is surrounded and protected by the bones of the spinal column. Unstable injuries of the spinal column, such as fractures or dislocation, can easily injure the cord. Spinal-cord injuries are usually permanent, but recovery is sometimes possible with careful treatment.

▶ *Field Assessment and Treatment of Spinal Cord Injury:* This is essentially the same as that for spine fracture, which is covered along with other fractures in the Musculoskeletal System chapter (page 117). Even if the cord is already injured, careful extrication, treatment, and evacuation controls further damage and increases the chance of recovery.

PERIPHERAL NERVES

The peripheral nervous system encompasses all nervous tissue outside of the brain and spinal cord. Peripheral nerves have the same cable-like structure as the spinal cord, but they are not enclosed in bony protection. They are damaged in the same manner as the cord by direct trauma from adjacent bones and joints which are unstable.

Peripheral nerves are also affected by pressure which can deprive them of adequate perfusion by oxygenated blood. "Backpacker's palsy" is the gradual onset of tingling and numbness of the arms caused by pressure on the nerves under the pack straps in the armpit and shoulder.

Assessment of Peripheral Nerve Injury: Loss of movement and sensation in the area beyond the site of an injury site can indicate nerve damage, for which little can be done in the field. However, remember that this can be caused by ischemia (loss of circulation), which is usually easily remedied.

Treatment of Peripheral Nerve Injury: In the field, the treatment of peripheral nerve injury is the same as the treatment for loss of circulation. Both are managed by removing the source of pressure, such as by loosening a splint, realigning a fracture or dislocation, or reducing swelling of an injured extremity. This is generic fracture management and is covered in the Musculoskeletal System Chapter.

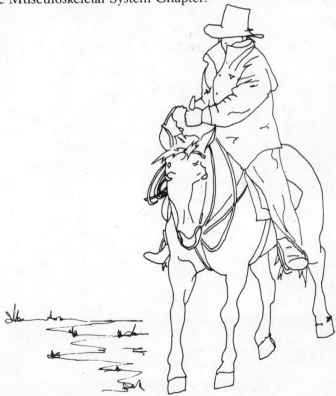

BONES,
JOINTS,
AND
SOFT TISSUE

7

THE MUSCULOSKELETAL

SYSTEM

After giving the X-rays one last look I noted my final diagnosis on the chart: "Mildly displaced fracture of the distal radius." What this really means is "broken wrist" and the patient needs to see an orthopedic surgeon. Of course, she knew that when the accident happened three days ago.

Karen was rock climbing above Chimney Pond on the North Face of Katahdin when a toe hold pulled loose, dropping her six feet onto a small ledge. Her partner, Steve, immediately took up the slack in the rope, and looked up to see if Karen needed further help.

She had landed on her right wrist and felt a crack and immediate pain, but a minute or two passed while Karen checked her position and equipment before she was able to assess her own injuries. Her wrist hurt, felt swollen, and her fingers were

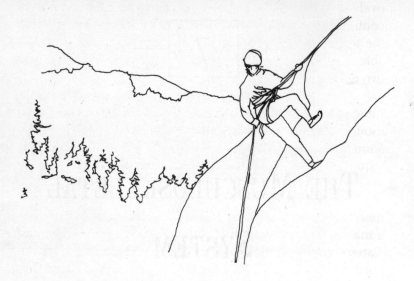

numb. She had no other apparent injuries and her partner was able to lower her to the ground.

Steve conducted a patient survey and found that Karen was alert, fully oriented and had no neck pain or tenderness. He noted the deformed and sore right wrist, but continued his exam to be sure that it was the only injury. He used gentle traction to restore bone position and a splint was fashioned using an aluminum stay from a backpack and a length of webbing for a sling. After a brief rest, the two climbers hiked back to the cabin.

As she warmed up, the return of normal color and sensation to Karen's fingers showed good blood perfusion beyond the injury. Even though she was pretty uncomfortable, and sometimes lightheaded and nauseated for the next several hours, Karen knew that this was no emergency.

There was no mechanism of injury which could cause volume shock. Her feeling faint was part of a normal, and harmless, acute stress reaction to the event. The splint effectively stabilized the wrist, and elevation and cold compresses controlled the swelling and pain. They continued to monitor the fingers to ensure circulation remained normal, and were able to safely wait out the storm which closed in for the next two days.

These two climbers recognized that this wrist injury was more of a logistical problem than a medical emergency, even though they knew it was probably fractured. Applying good common sense and basic understanding of the problem, they required neither rescue nor national news coverage.

Musculoskeletal injuries such as this are the most common backcountry medical problems. Although they are often a major inconvenience, they are rarely emergencies. Contrast Karen's story with the rescue of a teenaged girl in the mountains of Wyoming. During the traverse of a scree slope, a falling rock crushed the end of one of her fingers. She became extremely anxious, lightheaded and pale. The trip leader decided that she was in "shock" and called for helicopter evacuation. The aircraft made an emergency flight in bad weather, and the patient was "saved." Although it was very exciting and makes a great story, the risk to the helicopter and crew was totally unjustified.

You will recall from the previous chapters that a life-or-limb-threatening emergency involves a major problem with the Neurological, Respiratory, or Circulatory System. It is extremely important to recognize these problems when they occur. However, in the backcountry, it can be just as important to recognize when they don't.

If you've taken a first-aid course you may recall a lot of concern over fractures of the femur (thigh bone), skull, spine, pelvis, and ribs. It is important to realize here that the real problems are not the fractured bones themselves, but the potential injury to the vital organs next to them. Trauma patients do not die of fractures, sprains, strains, and contusions. They die from airway obstruction, blood loss, and brain injury.

With a fractured femur or pelvis, we actually worry more

about lacerated arteries (major Circulatory System injury). With the ribs we are concerned with the lungs, liver, or spleen (Circulatory and Respiratory system). And with the skull or spine fractures, it is the brain and spinal cord (Neurological system) inside that's of real concern.

Therefore, an important first step in handling any musculoskeletal problem is ruling out a major injury to one of the BIG 3 body systems. Remember, your primary survey should always focus on Airway, Breathing, Circulation, and Disability, not broken bones or dislocated joints. However, suspecting fractures in the pelvis, femur, spine, and skull should serve to focus your attention on the potential for BIG 3 problems.

If your Primary Survey discovers no existing BIG 3 injury, you have given yourself the luxury of time. Time to perform a secondary survey, think, treat, and safely evacuate yourself or your patient to medical care hours or days later. This may require help from rescue teams, but rarely as a hurried or risky undertaking.

STRUCTURE AND FUNCTION

Arms, legs, and fingers work on a system of cables, pulleys, and levers. The components are called muscles and tendons, ligaments, cartilage, and bones. The basic structure involves long bones connected by ligaments at joints which are padded by cartilage. Muscles and tendons work in balanced opposition across joints. The contraction of muscle on one side of the joint moves the bone one way, contraction on the other side moves it back. There are, of course, many types of bones and joints, but knowing each one is not required for effective field treatment.

The spine is best viewed as another long bone with the head and pelvis as joints on either end. The same basic parts and principles are at work. The major difference is the complexity and importance of the adjacent soft tissue.

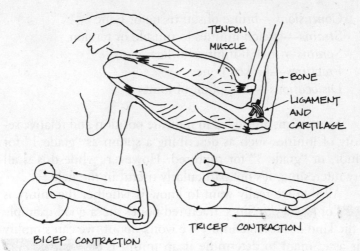

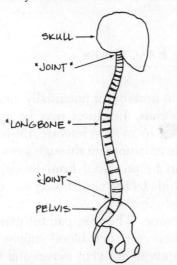

BICEP CONTRACTION

TRICEP CONTRACTION

Many muscles work in balanced opposition.

SKULL →

"JOINT"

"LONGBONE"

"JOINT"

PELVIS →

The spine can be considered a long bone with a joint at either end.

MUSCULOSKELETAL-SYSTEM PROBLEMS

The familiar medical terminology used to describe musculo-skeletal injury includes:

Contusions—bruise of soft tissue or bone
Strains—stretch injuries to muscle or tendon
Sprains—stretch injuries to ligaments
Fractures—broken bones
Dislocations—disruption of joints

More terms are added to indicate position and relative severity of injuries such as describing a sprain as "grade 1" for minor, or "grade 3" for ruptured. However, while this is all very interesting, it's not particularly useful in the field.

All that we really want to know is whether the injury is stable or unstable. Since fractured bones are a good example of the kind of unstable injury we worry about, we can simplify our assessment to determine if an injury is likely to involve fracture (unstable), or unlikely to involve fracture (stable).

FRACTURES

Fractured bones result in unstable or potentially unstable fragments with very sharp ends. Fractures may be open (compound) or closed (simple). In an open fracture, the fracture site is exposed to the outside environment through a wound in the skin. This opening can be produced from inside, by sharp bone ends, or from outside by the same object that caused the fracture.

Bones are living tissue. They are painful when injured and can bleed from their own rich blood supply. Unstable fragments can cause injury to adjacent nerves and blood vessels. It is important, therefore, to adequately stabilize any injury in which fracture is a possibility.

Since very few of us go backpacking or canoeing with an X-ray machine, it is often impossible to tell if a bone is actually broken. In the field, we use other assessment skills and rules of treatment. When an injury has the mechanism, signs, and symptoms of fracture, we treat it as such. For our purposes in the field:

> ### POSSIBLE FRACTURE = FRACTURE

In talking about the assessment and treatment of fractures we will consider three main groups;

1. *Extremity Fractures* requiring the stabilization of an individual extremity such as an arm or ankle.
2. *Dislocations* which may require reduction (putting the dislocated bone back in place) as part of the stabilization.
3. *Spine, Pelvis, and Femur Fractures* requiring stabilization of the whole body.

EXTREMITY FRACTURE

Mechanism Of Injury: Fractures of extremities can be caused by a variety of mechanisms reflecting the different ways force can be applied to the bone. The injury may be caused by leverage, twisting, direct impact, or a piece of bone being pulled away where the tendon or ligament attaches to it (avulsion fracture). For field purposes, however, defining mechanism of injury can be generalized to a yes-or-no question: was there sufficient force to cause a fracture?

I know what's coming next . . . "so what's sufficient force?" You're going to tell me about your Aunt Mable who broke her hip just stepping off a curb. You'll mention your friend who limped around on "stress fractures" for weeks before being diagnosed, and he didn't fall or anything. So, I agree with you, "sufficient force" can be difficult to define.

Positive Mechanism of Injury = Sufficient Force for Fracture
    Yes—A six-foot fall onto a ledge while rock climbing
    No—Waking up sore all over after a night sleeping on a
        ledge while rock climbing

Assessment of Extremity Fracture: To the vague definition of "sufficient force," we add the not-so-vague signs and symptoms of fracture. Combined with mechanism of injury, these provide a fairly clear guideline for identifying injuries that are likely to involve broken bones or other unstable components such as severe sprains.

POSITIVE MECHANISM + POSITIVE SIGNS AND SYMPTOMS = FRACTURE

Positive Signs and Symptoms

—The inability to move, use, or bear weight within an hour of the injury.

—The immediate development of severe pain, tenderness, and swelling.

—A history of feeling or hearing a "snap or crack."

—Obvious deformity or angulation.

—The sensation of bones grating against each other (crepitus) on movement.

—The patient or examiner feels instability of bones or joints. For example: "After the fall, I tried to ski but my knee gave out . . ."

Treatment of Extremity Fracture: An extremity fracture *by itself* is never an emergency. Our real concern is the potential for damage to the Circulatory and Nervous System tissues around the fracture site. The usual cause, and biggest worry, is extremity ischemia. However, treating the fracture correctly will often fix or prevent this problem.

The causes of extremity ischemia should sound familiar—either too little perfusion pressure in the Circulatory System, or too much pressure in the tissues to allow perfusion to occur. This can happen at the site of deformed fractures and dislocations where blood vessels are kinked or lacerated. Blood flow can also be stopped by splints or bandages which are tied too tight.

As we've said, Nervous System tissue is the most sensitive to oxygen deprivation. With the loss of effective blood circulation, peripheral nerves stop functioning and the extremity goes numb. With further obstruction, control of movement is lost as well.

The acronym we use for assessing this is CSM, which abbreviates Circulation, Sensation, and Movement. You have experienced problems with CSM if you've slept on your arm, or left it draped over a theater seat for too long. Circulation is impaired, it goes numb, and you can't move it. As circulation is restored, movement returns, then tingling, then full sensation.

Circulation is assessed by looking for evidence of blood flow in the injured extremity. Can you detect any pulses beyond ("distal" to) an area of injury? Is the skin normal in color, or pale or blue? Is the skin colder than the same extremity on the other side?

Sensation is the most important assessment tool. Loss of sensation is the first sign of ischemia. A normal patient will be able to feel the light touch of a finger or small object. In the early stages, the patient may complain of a tingling sensation, then numbness.

Movement refers to the patient's ability to move the extremity on command. The loss of the ability to move, such as wiggling fingers or toes, develops later in ischemia than the loss of sensation.

It is not unusual for an extremity to feel numb or cold immediately following injury, especially if the fracture results in deformity or the patient is having an Acute Stress Reaction. However, your treatment will usually result in a significant improvement in CSM status as circulation is restored.

As a general rule, extremity tissue can survive up to two hours of ischemia with minimal damage. Beyond this, the risk of permanent damage increases quickly with time. *If your treatment efforts do not succeed in restoring CSM, you have a limb-threatening emergency. Immediate evacuation is indicated if conditions permit.*

The generic treatment of fracture has three distinct phases:

1.   Traction Into Position (TIP)
2.   Hand Stable
3.   Splint Stable

1. Traction Into Position: Injured bones and joints, and the soft tissues around them, are much more comfortable and much less likely to be damaged further if splinted in normal anatomic position. While many injured extremities will remain in good position or return there on their own, some will require help from you.

We know that the idea of manipulating fractures contradicts older first-aid teaching, which states "splint it where it lies." But remember that older first-aid texts were not written from the perspective of the wilderness traveler. In fact, realigning deformed parts is fast becoming standard first-aid practice in all settings.

To restore anatomic position of a fractured bone we first apply Traction. Traction separates bone ends and reduces pain. Then, while traction is maintained, Position is restored. To understand how this works, picture moving a chain as a unit by holding the links under tension, rather than allowing them to rattle against each other.

Shaft fractures of long bones are brought into the line of normal bone axis, the "in line" position. This is where the effect of opposing muscles is most balanced, and the blood circulation to the extremity beyond the injury is best maintained. If you're not sure what the realigned extremity should look like, check the other side. Isn't it fortunate that people have two of almost everything?

Fractured joints, such as elbows, shoulders, and knees, usually do not need to be repositioned. If your patient is con-

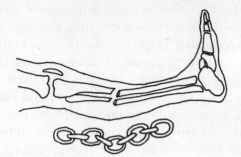

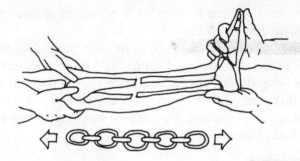

*Hand stable—prevents further damage from sharp
bone fragments until splint can be applied.*

scious and mobile, he will have already found the most comfortable position for the injured joint and be holding it there by
the time you come along. If not, gentle TIP to a position in
the mid-range of the joint's normal motion is the best approach for long-term care.

In severely deformed joints, such as dislocations, there is
likely to be a loss of circulation, sensation, and movement
(CSM) beyond the injury site. Under these conditions, TIP
with movement toward the mid-range position is used until
circulation is re-established. In some specific cases, which
we'll discuss later, TIP can be used to reduce dislocations (put
the dislocated bone back in place) with a significant improvement in comfort and circulation.

Traction Into Position is a safe procedure if done properly. It generally decreases pain rather than increases it. However, to be successful it helps to have the cooperation and
confidence of the injured person. Pulling on a fractured leg
without telling it's owner how or why you're going to do it
won't win you any friends. If necessary, you and your assistants may want to practice on an uninjured limb first.

Occasionally it will be impossible to comfortably and
safely restore position, even using TIP. *You should discontinue
TIP and stabilize the injury in the position found if TIP causes
a significant increase in pain, or if movement of the extremity
is prevented by resistance.*

Open shaft fractures with bone ends protruding through
the skin are still managed with TIP. Bone ends are often
pulled beneath the skin surface when traction is applied. It is
best, however, to first clean the exposed bone by irrigating
with water and brushing away debris (see Chapter 8 section on
High Risk Wounds, page 133).

Hand Stable: Once you have repositioned an extremity injury, stability must be maintained until the splint can take
over. This may mean having someone hold gentle traction on
the extremity while you collect materials. If you don't have an
army of assistants you may have to use snow, rocks, or pieces
of equipment to hold things in place. The important thing is,
don't just let the foot, arm, or whatever lay there unsupported
now that you've got it where you want it. Of course, if you
were really thinking, you might have had your splint materials
ready *before* you started the process.

Splint Stable: Splinting is the real art of first aid. We've seen
an incredible variety of splints from fabulously expensive
stainless-steel jobs with dozens of moving parts, to disorganized collections of firewood and baling twine. The best of
them, however, are simple, effective, and probably in your
backpack or canoe right now. Any splint will be good when it
meets the General Principles of Splinting, no matter what its
components are in real life.

GENERAL PRINCIPALS OF SPLINTING

1. Long Bone Fractures—Splint in the "in-line" (looks normal) position.

2. Long Bone Fractures—Include the joint above and below the injury. For example, to effectively splint a lower leg fracture, the ankle and knee must be immobilized.

3. Joint Fractures—Splint in the position found, or in the mid-range position.

4. Joint Fractures—Include the bones above and below. For example: to splint the elbow, the forearm and upper arm are included in the splint. There is no need to include adjacent joints in the splint. The shoulder and wrist may be left mobile.

5. Splints should be well padded. This allows normal bone and joint contours to fit your splint material without pressure points or loose spots.

6. Multi-dimensional splints are best. This is where splint material is applied on both sides of the injured part and generally provides the best stability and comfort.

7. Splints should be strong and snug enough to prevent movement of the injured parts.

8. Monitor splints frequently—Pain is a good indicator of movement. Bone fragments are adequately stabilized if the pain is well controlled. Check distal (beyond the injury) circulation, sensation, and movement (CSM) before and after splinting. Continue to monitor CSM, especially during prolonged transport. This should be done every fifteen minutes in the first few hours, then at least every hour thereafter. This is especially important during cold weather because extremity ischemia can result in frostbite.

The splint should allow easy access to fingertips or toes for monitoring. If ischemia develops, you may need to loosen or rearrange the splint. Your splint should improve and preserve blood circulation and nerve function, not impair it. A good splint should provide decreased pain and intact CSM.

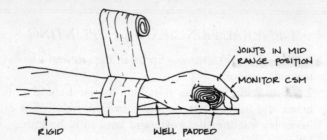

Hand, wrist, and forearm splint

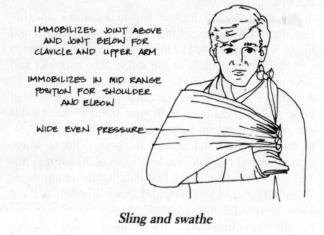

Sling and swathe

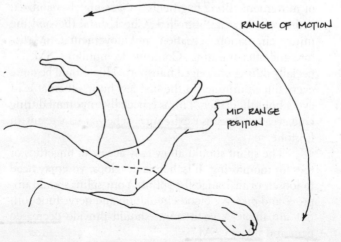

Range of motion of elbow.

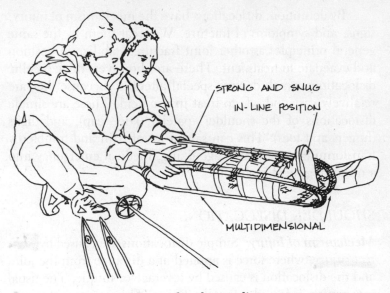

STRONG AND SNUG
IN-LINE POSITION

MULTIDIMENSIONAL

Lower leg, knee splint

Once the extremity is stabilized with your perfect splint, and you are satisfied that CSM is improving, treatment should include rest and elevation to reduce swelling and discomfort (see Treatment of Stable Injuries, page 125). As long as distal CSM remains normal, or continues to improve, you can take your time planning a safe and comfortable evacuation.

JOINT DISLOCATIONS

The average garden-variety joint is a complex, mobile assembly of bones, ligaments, cartilage, tendon and muscle. To the delight of orthopedic surgeons everywhere, these structures can be injured in a wide variety of combinations and levels of severity. A dislocation occurs when enough force is applied to the bone to tear the restraining ligaments and allow the joint to come apart.

By definition, dislocations have the mechanism of injury, signs, and symptoms of fracture. We treat them by the same general principles as other joint fracture; stabilize in position and evacuate to treatment. There are, however, three specific dislocations which deserve special attention because they are relatively easy and safe to treat in the field. These are simple dislocations of the shoulder, patella (knee cap), and digits (fingers and toes). This can save a lot of pain and trouble by transforming a gruesome, agonizing, medical emergency into a minor logistical problem.

SHOULDER DISLOCATIONS

Mechanism of Injury: Simple dislocations are caused by *indirect injury*, where force is applied at a distance from the joint and the dislocation is caused by leverage or torque. The usual mechanism is forced external rotation. This movement is similar to throwing a baseball, high bracing with a kayak paddle, or catching a fall on an outstretched arm while skiing. Fractures are uncommon, and generally do not interfere with treatment.

These injuries can be extremely uncomfortable and result in significant damage to the joint and surrouding soft tissue if untreated for more than a couple of hours. Fortunately these dislocations can often be reduced using gentle TIP even by an inexperienced rescuer. This is best accomplished within an hour of the injury, before severe swelling and muscle spasm occur.

The more serious dislocation from *direct injury* is usually the result of a high-speed impact into a solid object. Distinguishing this mechanism from that of indirect force is usually not difficult. Sufficient force is applied directly to the joint area to force the bone ends apart. These injuries are almost always associated with other major injury, and probably will not be your primary focus of attention in those cases.

Assessment of Shoulder Dislocation: Assessment is directed toward identifying the simple dislocations caused by indirect force which may be fixed in the field. This is where careful attention to the mechanism of injury during your surveys and history can really pay off.

The patient will describe the classic mechanism of injury consistent with simple dislocation. He will frequently give a history of recurrent dislocation in the same extremity. On exam, you'll notice right away that the person with a dislocated shoulder is in moderate to severe discomfort. There is often some degree of Acute Stress Reaction. In about half the cases there is some CSM impairment of the arm and hand. The shoulder itself loses the rounded contour and becomes a "step-off deformity" and has a hollow area where the shoulder is normally full and rounded (see illustration). The patient will be unwilling to move the shoulder joint without help and coaching.

Occasionally, a shoulder dislocation can be confused with a shoulder *separation.* A separation refers to disruption of the joint between the distal end of the clavicle and the scapula (AC joint). The usual mechanism of injury is a direct blow to the top of the shoulder during a fall.

This joint lies directly above the shoulder joint and can have a similar "step-off" appearance when injured. The key difference is that, in separation, the shoulder joint and upper arm remain mobile. In dislocation, mobility is lost.

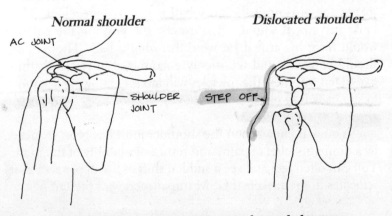

Normal shoulder   *Dislocated shoulder*

AC JOINT

SHOULDER JOINT   STEP OFF

A dislocated shoulder loses its normal rounded contour.

REDUCTION

➡ **Treatment of Shoulder Dislocation:** The simple dislocation of the shoulder should generally be treated in the field if the evacuation time to definitive care will be greater than two hours. It should also be considered if the evacuation will be exceptionally difficult or dangerous to perform while the shoulder remains displaced. These criteria probably apply to most backcountry and marine situations.

Several techniques are effective in reducing dislocated shoulders. Traction and external rotation, the most effective and easiest to perform in the field, requires only a small patch of level ground and one rescuer. Remember, before starting, to check and document distal CSM. You will want to be sure that your treatment has resulted in improvement.

To begin, the patient's arm is supported while he is moved so that he lies on his back. Gentle TIP on the upper arm will help relieve pain during movement. The patient's co-operation and relaxation is essential. This will take some time; there is no reason to torture your patient with speed. Once the patient is lying on his back, the rescuer applies gentle traction to the arm and slowly swings it into a postion about 90 degrees from the body, with the elbow bent.

The rescuer continues to hold TIP with one hand just above the elbow. Traction should be firm, but not enough to slide the patient across the ground. With the other hand on the patient's forearm, the rescuer gently and slowly externally rotates the arm until the "baseball position" is reached. This looks just like it sounds. It is exactly the position the patient would have his arm if he were throwing a ball. The patient should be gently and repeatedly encouraged to relax. Within five to ten minutes, the muscles will fatigue, allowing the joint to slip back into place. Remember to stop this process if pain or resistance is increased!

You will know when the shoulder joint has been reduced by a dramatic relief of pain, and return of mobility of the joint. You can often feel and see a sudden shift of the upper arm as it relocates in the socket. If CSM impairment was present before

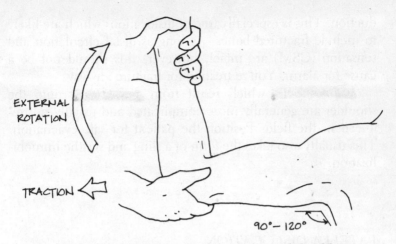

EXTERNAL
ROTATION

TRACTION

90° – 120°

Baseball position for reducing a dislocated shoulder

reduction, it will rapidly improve afterward. Remember to check and document CSM both before and after reduction.

Following reduction, your patient usually experiences significant relief and will thank you profusely enough to become embarrassing. At this point it is worth remembering that a joint dislocation has the positive mechanism, signs, and symptoms of fracture and should be treated as such. Inevitably, swelling will occur and pain will increase over time. The most effective splint is a simple sling and swathe or the equivalent.

An alternative reduction technique is Simple Hanging Traction. This is accomplished by stabilizing the patient face down on the edge of a flat ledge or deck where the dislocated arm can hang straight down. Pad the axillae (arm pit). Ten to fifteen pounds of weight can then be taped or tied to the arm to apply steady gravitational traction. As the patient ultimately fatigues and relaxes, the shoulder will slip back into place. This technique may take up to sixty minutes to be successful.

Some shoulders will remain painful immediately after reduction. This is especially true of dislocations which are likely to include fractured bones. As long as distal circulation and sensation (CSM) are intact, however, this should not be a cause for alarm. You're treating for fracture anyway.

Dislocations which result from direct force onto the shoulder are generally more complicated and usually not reduced in the field. Position the patient for safe evacuation. This usually also takes the form of a sling and swathe immobilization.

PATELLA DISLOCATION

Mechanism of Injury: The patella (kneecap) is an isolated bone imbedded as a kind of fulcrum in the quadriceps tendon. This large tendon transmits the powerful force of the quadriceps muscle in the front of the thigh to the front of the lower leg to allow you to extend the knee. This is the motion you'd use to bring your foot forward to kick a ball, or kick your climbing partner for dropping you.

The quadriceps tendon passes over and through a groove in the femur, like a cable through a pulley. In patellar dislocation, the cable, patella included, slips off the femur making it impossible for the knee to function.

Like the shoulder, the patella can dislocate with a direct blow (rare) or indirect mechanism, typically a sudden extension of the knee. The patient often has a history of recurrent dislocation. The dislocation is always lateral (to the outside), leaving the patella pinned against the outside of the knee by the pull of the quadriceps.

Assessment of Patella Dislocation: The appearance can be deceiving. Shifting the patella laterally will make the bony prominence on the inside of the knee stand out and look like

the missing patella. Don't be fooled. Feel for the patella laterally and you'll find it.

Like the shoulder, these dislocations also are extremely
uncomfortable and there is little or no motion of the joint possible. Distal circulation and sensation is usually unaffected,
but you should check it anyway. Damage to surrounding soft
tissue will increase with time, as will the difficulty of reduction.

Treatment of Patella Dislocation: Like the shoulder, a dislocated patella should be reduced if the evacuation time will be
greater than two hours, or the evacuation will be unreasonably
difficult. Reducing a dislocated patella is also reversing the
mechanim of injury. Take the tension off the "cable" by
straightening the knee and flexing the hip (have the patient sit
up) and then pop the patella back in place with your thumbs.
Relief and profuse thanks will result, but splint the knee for
fracture anyway. These injuries are unstable and will result in
significant pain and swelling after several hours. Again, remember to check and document CSM status before and after
reduction.

DIGIT DISLOCATION—FINGERS AND TOES

Mechanism of Injury: Joints in the fingers usually dislocate
due to an indirect force which levers the bone ends apart. The
classic example is catching a falling soft ball the wrong way.
Other examples include catching a disappearing canoe wrong,
catching a falling climber wrong, or just having your hand in
the wrong place at the wrong time. In any case, what you end
up with is a finger pointing the wrong way at the distal (DIP)
or middle (PIP) joint.

There is often an associated small chip fracture. Motion

of the joint is usually impossible, and there will be some degree of CSM impairment. Damage will increase with time.

➡ **Treatment of Digit Dislocation:** Your first reaction when confronted with a dislocated finger will be to want it back where it belongs, especially if it is yours. Fortunately this is exactly what should be done if definitive care will be delayed more than two hours. TIP is the same as for shaft fractures, in the normal axis of the digit. Reduction will be most easily accomplished right after the injury has occurred before pain and swelling become significant.

After getting your patient's consent, simply grasp the end of the offending finger with one hand, and the rest of the finger in the other. Pull the end of the finger first in the direction it is pointing, then while maintaining traction swing it back in line. This is not easy as it sounds, but it does work. You'll probably need to wrap the end of your patient's finger in gauze or a bandanna to help keep your grip.

After reduction, resist the temptation to play with it. Remember, fracture is very likely and it will need medical attention at some point. So splint it in the mid-range of the joint's motion and give it a rest. Again, don't forget to check CSM before and after reduction. Things should improve with your treatment.

Difficult Dislocations: In the backcountry any dislocation which resists your efforts at reduction can become a serious problem. Pain may be severe, and the potential for soft tissue damage increases with time. If CSM is significantly impaired, and cannot be restored by traction and repositioning, immediate evacuation to medical care is warranted. These are limb-threatening emergencies.

Spine, Femur, and Pelvis Fractures

In stabilizing musculoskeletal injuries to the spine, pelvis, and femur, we apply the same assessment skills and splinting principles as in extremity fractures. However to satisfy these principles, the splint is usually a long backboard or litter which can secure the hips, back and neck. This pretty well eliminates walking your patient out of the woods.

The equipment necessary is brought to the scene by rescue teams or aircraft, and requires a carry-out or airlift evacuation. Your role will usually be limited to moving the patient to shelter, or shelter to the patient, and stabilizing in place until help arrives.

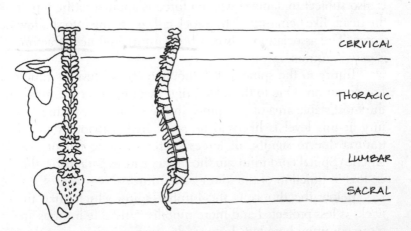

Anatomic divisions of the spine

SPINE FRACTURES

Mechanism of Injury: The spine is fractured like any other bone, by both direct and indirect trauma. All spine injury is significant, but the most potentially devastating is the fracture or dislocation of the cervical spine (neck).

The delicate tissue of the spinal cord, really an extension of the brain, is surrounded and protected by the bones of the spinal column. Unstable injuries of the bony spinal column can easily injure the cord. Cord injury above the level of the third vertebrae in the neck will cause respiratory arrest. Below that level, injuries usually result in quadriplegia, that is, loss of function to all four extremities. These injuries are usually permanent, but recovery is sometimes possible with careful treatment.

The neck is the most commonly injured area because it is the most mobile section of the spine, linking the heavy mass of the head with the body. As a result it is very prone to injury which snaps the head back and forth like a ball on a string. It is also subject to damage when a force is applied to the top of the head, like being struck by a rock fall, or diving into shallow water. The association between head injury and neck fracture is very common.

Injury to the spine at the thoracic (chest) level is much less common. Due to the added rigidity of the rib cage, this is the most stable area of the spine. In the wilderness setting, injury at this level is likely to be associated with other major trauma due to significant forces such as a long fall or avalanche. Spinal cord injury in the thorax causes paraplegia; that is, loss of function of the lower extremities.

Below the thorax is the lumbar spine which, like the neck, is less protected and more mobile. Unstable injuries are more common here but, fortunately, cord injury is rare. Near the top of the lumbar spine, the spinal cord separates into individual nerve roots which looks like a loose bundle of linguini. These nerve roots are much more mobile and less likely to be injured.

Assessment of Spine Fracture: Assessment of spine fracture is similar to that of other fractures, but there are important differences because the consequences of spinal-cord injury are so devastating. We tend to be much more conservative in our assessment and treatment.

In the urban setting, ambulance crews routinely immobilizes any trauma patient with a positive mechanism of injury for spine fracture. This works fine in situations where the patient will arrive at the hospital within a few minutes. The full assessment can be carried out in the controlled environment of the Emergency Department. In the backcountry, however, we must recognize that committing a patient and rescuers to full spinal immobilization and evacuation can be impractical, and even dangerous. Our field assessment must be more complete.

In the presence of a positive mechanism of injury we look for the same signs and symptoms of fracture used in extremity injury. We apply the same principle: Possible fracture = Fracture. But, since the brain and spinal cord may be involved, we must consider the possibility that normal body reactions, such as feeling pain, may be absent. This is especially true when spinal injury is accompanied by head injury. Therefore, a critical part of your assessment has to do with the reliability of your own exam.

In cases where the patient is not alert, is intoxicated, or altered in mental status, your examination for signs of spine fracture will be unreliable. You must assume that the spine is fractured and treat it as such, even when your examination is negative. You can evaluate again later when your patient may have cleared his head, calmed down, or sobered up. In the backcountry this could happen before you leave camp to get help, or at any time during the evacuation.

If, however, you can determine that your patient is calm, cooperative, sober, and alert, your examination can be considered reliable. If there are no signs and symptoms of fracture, you can be comfortable in your assessment of "no spine fracture." There is no need for spinal immobilization.

➡️ *Treatment of Spine Fracture:* For field purposes, the spine is treated as a long bone with a joint at each end. The positioning and treatment principles are the same. The techniques will vary depending on the equipment available, the terrain to be crossed, and the people doing it.

Use Traction Into Position to restore the injured spine to the normal anatomic position. As with other long bones, it will be most stable and least likely to injure adjacent nerves and blood vessels. The normal in-line position is also best for airway protection.

Hand stable for the spine involves maintaining the alignment of the bone throughout any lifting, rolling, or carrying.

FIELD ASSESSMENT OF SPINE FRACTURES

In the presence of a Positive or Uncertain Mechanism of Injury

Positive Signs and Symptoms = Spine Fracture

Unreliable Exam = Spine Fracture

Reliable Exam + Negative Signs and Symptoms

= No Spine Fracture

Unreliable Exam	*Reliable Exam*
ASR with pain masking	Calm
Combative or Confused	Cooperative
Intoxicated	Sober
Altered Consciousness	Alert

Positive Signs and Symptoms
1. Pain in the spine.
2. Tenderness of the spine when palpated.
3. Abnormal motor or sensory function of the extremities.

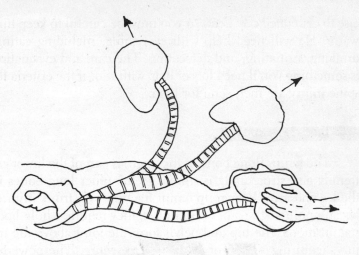

Traction into position (TIP) for spine stabilization.

Traction is maintained on the head until the spine is *Splint stable*. The head and neck are secured by a collar, and the splint is completed by the long board or litter which immobilizes the lower spine and pelvis.

As you can imagine, this is not often easy. In most cases where you cannot prove that the spine is not injured, you will be better off setting up camp right where you are and awaiting a better exam, or rescue. If staying put is not an option, you should provide the maximum stability possible to the spine before movement. Carrying the patient supine on his back in an improvised litter is best. Having a person with an injured back or neck walk themselves to shelter should be an absolute last resort.

For short moves or stabilization while waiting for help you can use a combination of improvised collar and short spine board. A section of ensolite sleeping pad or rolled tarp can be an effective cervical collar. A snowshoe or pack frame can double as a short spine board. As with extremity injuries, snow, rocks or equipment can be placed around a supine patient to prevent movement.

The long-term care of the spine-injured patient is difficult, especially outdoors. The patient will be unable to exercise to generate body heat, so you must be careful to keep him warm. He will need help with everything, including eating, drinking, urinating, and defecating. The care and evacuation is something you'll need lots of help with. So, if the criteria for spine injury are met, send for help.

FEMUR FRACTURE

The femur (long bone in the thigh) is part of the lower extremity and structurally is similar to the other long bones in the leg and arm. We group femur fracture with trunk injuries because, unlike the other extremities, they require whole-body stabilization. The hip and pelvis form the joint above the injury, requiring a litter or backboard to secure. The powerful thigh muscles are easily thrown into spasm by movement.

They also deserve separate consideration due to the possibility of volume shock from a lacerated femoral artery (circulatory system injury). It is not easy to fracture a femur. Massive direct force is required.

Assessment of Femur Fracture: Of the signs and symptoms of fracture, the one most typical of the femur is severe pain. Unless there is pain masking from other injury or intoxication, these patients will be very uncomfortable. They do not smile, laugh, or ask questions. They hurt. Movement is difficult, and weight bearing is impossible. If the injured person (without pain masking) looks at all comfortable, you have reason to doubt that the femur is fractured.

Suspected femur fracture should lead you to observe for signs of volume shock from major Circulatory System injury. Even in a closed fracture of the femur, considerable blood can be lost into the thigh. Massive swelling will often be evident. The *primary* problem may be a fractured femur, but the more serious *anticipated problem* is volume shock.

➡ *Treatment of Femur Fracture:* Firm Traction Into Position reduces pain and spasm, reduces the chance of injury to arteries and nerves, and reduces the space available inside the thigh for blood loss. TIP should be applied as soon as possible whenever femur fracture is recognized, and maintained throughout the splinting process.

The ideal femur splint would maintain traction all the way to the hospital, and there are several types of specialized traction splints made for this purpose. These splints require training and experience to use and, even when properly applied, can impair circulation. This quickly becomes a problem in the long-term care situation.

Improvised traction splints for field use employing ski poles, canoe paddles and other pieces of equipment are usually more architecturally interesting than medically useful. The simplest, safest, and most universal splint is firm immobilization on a long board or litter without traction.

PELVIC FRACTURES

Mechanism of Injury: Like the femur, it takes a significant force to fracture the pelvis. These are usually the injuries of long falls, high-speed ski accidents, and avalanches. There are, however, rare instances when the pelvis can be fractured by a seemingly mild event. Also, like the femur, a major concern is the possibility of severe bleeding from arteries and veins adjacent to the fracture site.

Assessment of Pelvic Fractures: Pelvic fractures are a little tricky. They are usually quite painful, but not always. They can also be difficult to distinguish from hip or lower lumbar spine fractures. There are no single outstanding signs or symptoms. In the presence of positive mechanism, pelvic pain and tenderness, and inability to bear weight, you have little choice but to treat for fracture.

Treatment of Pelvic Fractures: Pelvic fracture also requires immobilization of the trunk to meet the principles of splinting. Because of danger to adjacent blood vessels, possible pelvic fractures deserve long board or litter stabilization also. Volume shock should be in your anticipated problem list, if it's not already present. As with the femur, it is often going to be best to stabilize in place and call for help with evacuation.

STABLE INJURIES

Just before Karen's arrival in the clinic, we discharged a patient with a knee injury. He left the same way he had arrived, walking. Paul had been skiing the snowfields above King Pine chair yesterday when he caught a ski tip on a tree, twisting the lower leg outward. He felt mild pain in the right knee, but was able to continue skiing for several more hours.

He felt no pop or snap at the time of injury, and no instability afterwards. It was not until later in the evening that the pain and swelling began. He soaked in the hot tub for an hour and went to bed.

Today Paul's knee is very sore. There is slight swelling and tenderness on the inside of the joint. There is good range of motion, but with considerable pain. Even with these findings today, however, the history indicates that the injury does not reflect positive signs and symptoms of fracture. Paul has a stable injury.

The treatment for Paul's injury is **R**est, **I**ce, **E**levation, and **C**ompression (RICE). After a day or so Paul can return to whatever activity he can do without causing significant pain (Pain-Free Activity). He should be ready to ski again within a week or so.

Assessment of Stable Injuries: Typical signs and symptoms of stable injury include positive mechanism and pain, but *none of the specific signs and symptoms of fracture* (see page 102). The patient is able to use, move, or bear weight more or less normally within the first hour following injury. There is no history of a "snap, crack, or pop." There is no deformity, crepitus (grating sound), or sense of instability.

Swelling is common, but develops slowly over several hours from the accumulation of edema fluid, rather than rapidly from bleeding. It is not unusual for the patient to experience considerable pain and immobility the next day as this swelling reaches its peak. This is especially true if he continued to use the injured part for a while after the injury.

Treatment of Stable Injuries: The early treatment of stable injuries is essentially the same as for fracture. This conservative treatment prevents the development of disability from excessive pain and swelling.

RICE

R = Rest. Local rest—splinted or limited use.
I = Ice. Cold packs. Use as tolerated first twenty-four hours.
C = Compression, i.e., ACE bandage. Use only on distal extremity.
E = Elevation. Raise the injury above heart level.

Pain-Free Activity (PFA): After the first twenty-four hours, or when most of the pain and swelling has resolved, the injured person may perform whatever activity is possible as long as additional pain is not caused. This may include skiing, or it may require very limited use around camp for several days.

Medication: Anti-inflammatory medication such as aspirin or ibuprofen can help reduce swelling and discomfort.

Remember the 24-hours swelling curve? Most of the swelling will occur over the first six hours. Afterward, the rate of swelling tapers off over the next eighteen hours. Little swelling generally occurs therafter. Elevation and Rest are the most important elements of RICE, and most useful early on while the swelling is likely to be the worst. Ice is also very helpful, if available. Even in the summer, you can achieve some cooling by evaporation by wrapping the injury in a water-soaked bandage.

Following these treatment guidelines, all stable injuries should show steady improvement. If not, your patient is being too active, or your assessment may be wrong. Never be afraid to reassess the situation and change your mind. Medical people do it all the time.

CASE STUDY

S: A 23-year-old female instructor glissading a snow field in the Tetons caught her heel in the snow, causing a tumbling fall. She felt a pop and a brief burning pain in her left knee. On attempting to stand, the knee "gave out." She did not hit her head, and has no neck pain. She has full memory of the event. She has an allergy to codeine, takes ibuprofen for headaches, has never injured the knee before, has no significant past medical history. Her last meal was 20 minutes ago. The glissade was at the end of a 10-day backcountry trip, with only a half mile to go.

O: The instructor was found sitting upright in stable position with the left knee flexed. She was fully alert, and warm and reasonably dry. She had no neck tenderness. The left knee was tender, but not swollen, deformed, or discolored. She was able to flex and extend the knee fully with little discomfort. Distal CSM was intact. There was no other obvious injury. Vital signs at 13:20 were normal.

A: Fracture left knee

P: The knee was splinted with a snowshoe, and an improvised litter was fashioned from ensolite pads and nylon webbing. The woman was carried the last half mile to the road. Distal CSM was monitored by asking her if she could feel and wiggle her toes inside her boots.

Discussion: Although the temptation to limp the last half mile was very strong, the patient agreed to the appropriate treatment. This injury fit the criteria for fracture because of the history of a "pop" during injury and the instability experienced afterwards. This story is typical of a ligament rupture, which is every bit as unstable as a fracture.

CASE STUDY

S: A 17-year-old girl caught her right index finger between loose rocks during a descent of a scree slope fifteen miles from the trailhead. She was able to dislodge herself, but complained of immediate pain. Shortly afterward, she became dizzy and nauseated. The group leader climbed back up to examine the girl. Witnesses told him that she did not fall, and was not struck by anything. She has no allergies, is not on medication, has no sigificant past medical history, and is up to date on tetanus vaccination. She had breakfast two hours ago. She had been walking without difficulty prior to the accident and was well rested and hydrated. The rock was stable but the weather was cool and windy.

O: The patient was found lying against a large rock. She was disoriented, pale, and sweaty. The tip of the right index finger is swollen and very tender with a superficial abrasion. There was no other injury. Her Vital Signs at 11:30 were—BP: unknown, P: 64, R: 24, Skin: pale, cool, moist, T: feels cool, C: V on AVPU with confusion and disorientation.

A: 1. Fracture tip of right index finger.
  2. Abrasion of right index finger.
  3. Acute Stress Reaction

A': 1. Infection of abrasion right index finger.

P: The finger was immersed in clean, cold water to irrigate the abrasion and relieve pain. She was encouraged to lie in a sleeping bag and calm down. Her Vital Signs, rechecked at 12:00, were normal. The finger was splinted by taping it to the third finger with a gauze pad and antibiotic ointment between the fingers.

The girl was instructed to keep the finger elevated as much as possible, and use cool soaks for swelling and pain relief during rest stops. The wound was to be irrigated, and the dressing changed daily. She was cautioned about the signs and symptoms of infection, and instructed to check circulation and sensation at the fingertip frequently. She would be referred to medical care when the group reached the road in three days.

Discussion: Although this patient was displaying very frightening signs and symptoms immediately after the injury, there was no mechanism to explain it, except ASR. The changes in Level of Consciousness and mental status rapidly resolved with rest, reassurance, and pain relief, leaving only an unhappy girl with a sore finger.

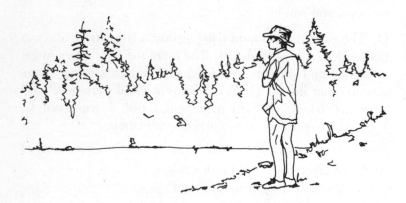

8

SKIN
AND SOFT TISSUE

Laceration of the skin is one of the most common reasons that Outward Bound students are evacuated from their solo experience at the Hurricane Island School. The wounds are almost always caused by a slip of the knife blade while rendering some indispensable tool or art form from a stubborn piece of driftwood. These injuries occur, not for lack of preparation and precaution, but rather because the creative spirit seems to get the better of the student's common sense.

To improve this situation, instructors have used every technique from giving detailed whittling lessons, to "no whittling" policies, to outright banning of knives. But I like the creative spirit, and believe the knife to be the most necessary of tools. Therefore, I tend to favor instruction and precaution, and a good talk on wound care.

Students carry into the field with them everything they need to care for minor wounds. This consists of their own two hands, fresh water, soap, and clean gauze dressings. Their primary goal is to assist the body's own defensive and healing mechanisms. Definitive care, like suturing (stitches) can be performed hours or days later if necessary.

STRUCTURE AND FUNCTION

The skin is the largest of the body's organs. It performs the remarkable function of separating the flora and fauna of the outside environment from the sterile, temperature- and chemical-sensitive internal organs. Most of the time it does a pretty good job, considering it's only about a quarter of an inch thick.

Soft tissue refers to the tissues between the skin and underlying bone, joints, and organs. It includes fat, muscle, and connective tissue as well as the small vessels and nerves found in these layers. Problems begin when the protective outer layer of skin is damaged, and the tissue beneath is exposed. This allows fungi, bacteria, and other creatures to invade unprotected tissue, as well as allowing vital body fluids to escape.

SKIN AND SOFT TISSUE PROBLEMS

WOUNDS

A wound is any injury that disrupts the skin. It can be superficial or deep. It can also involve structures other than soft tissue such as bone, major nerves and vessels, and internal organs. They come in a fascinating variety of types, but for field purposes we'll put them in four manageable groups:

Laceration and Avulsion: The skin is divided (laceration) or sliced or torn away (avulsion). They may be superficial or deep. There may be an "avulsion flap" still attached. The wound may also include some crushed and dead tissue.

Amputation: A complete segment of an extremity is lost, such as a finger or arm. Bleeding may be severe. The amputated part may sometimes be reattached several hours after injury.

Shallow Wounds: Superficial burns and abrasions can disrupt the skin, but not penetrate through into the soft tissue.

Puncture Wounds: Skin disruption is minmal, but the injury extends into the soft tissue. The object which causes the puncture drags bacteria and other foreign material into the wound, almost invariably causing some degree of infection.

All wounds damage blood vessels and cause bleeding. The body can stop this blood loss by automatically constricting blood vessels at the injury site to reduce flow. A clot then begins to form, and if left undisturbed, can bring bleeding to a halt within fifteen minutes. Serious bleeding problems can develop when injured vessels are numerous or very large. Severe blood loss (BIG 3 Circulatory System problem) can occur before the clotting mechanism seals the wound.

After the blood loss has been stopped, the slower process of wound repair begins. The initial stages of natural wound cleansing occur over a period of several days. The clot surface dries, forming a natural bandage in the form of a scab. Underlying tissue is further protected by the process of inflammation which forms a protective barrier below.

Any contamination, such as dirt and bacteria, is moved to the surface as the wound drains. By the third or fourth day, the protective barriers are established and cleansing is well underway. The signs of normal inflammation—redness, warmth, swelling, and pain—begin to subside as the protective barrier continues to grow stronger.

After six to eight days the wound is very resistant to new outside contamination. As inflammation subsides, wound edges migrate together and form a scar where they meet. Re-injury, or excessive movement of the wound area, during the early stages can disrupt the barrier effect, fostering infection and delayed healing.

If the inflammatory process is overwhelmed and the wound is not internally sealed or externally drained, invading bacteria may pass through the protective barrier into surrounding tissues. If the body's immune system is unable to control them, bacteria can reproduce rapidly, causing an infection. In an attempt to re-establish the barrier, the body increases local inflammation. Pus develops as the cellular debris and edema fluid accumulates. This combination of processes produce the early signs and symptoms of infection.

If the infection spreads, it will ultimately enter the general circulation and cause a systemic infection, sometimes called blood poisoning. The body responds with systemic inflammation, which produces a generalized redness, fever, and pain. Patients with systemic infection are very sick. Fortunately, this rarely happens as a complication of skin wounds in healthy individuals.

Some wounds are more prone to infection than others. These we label as "high risk" and require more care and earlier medical attention. These include puncture wounds and wounds involving joints and other complex structures. It also includes wounds which are dirty or involve crushed or dead tissue.

Assessment of Wounds: Although wounds, like fractures, are sometimes obvious and dramatic, they are rarely life-threatening in themselves. Assessment is directed initially toward finding and treating associated BIG 3 problems. Then, the wound itself is evaluated for evidence of "high risk" factors.

HIGH-RISK WOUNDS

Dirty Wounds—Injuries with imbedded foreign material such as gravel, sawdust, or clothing fibers, harbor bacteria which is difficult to dislodge.

Ragged Wounds—Wounds in which there is crushed, shredded, or dead tissue that provides a good growth medium for bacteria.

Underlying Injury—Wounds which involve injuries to joints, tendons, and bones (open fractures) are difficult to clean adequately and are prone to serious infection.

Bite Wounds—From humans or other animals. Mouths harbor a wide variety of virulent bugs. Human bites are among the worst. Cats are pretty bad, too. Any wound exposed to human or animal saliva constitutes a bite wound. Perhaps the most common example is the small laceration one can get across the knuckles of the hand when punching an opponent in the mouth. These have a very high infection rate.

Puncture Wounds—A small opening in the skin with a wound track that extends through several layers of tissue deposits bacteria in areas that are unable to drain properly. These have a way of looking minor at first, but becoming a big problem later. This is especially true of the "nail through the sneaker into the bottom of the foot" injuries.

Treatment of Soft-Tissue Wounds: Treat the BIG 3 problems first! Your riding partner goes over the handlebars on a steep descent and you find him sitting in the trail with his face covered with blood from a small scalp laceration. Your first instinct is to wipe the blood away and help him up because you hate the sight of blood and want everything to look normal again. This is a perfectly natural reaction, but dead wrong. Do not forget that this is the mechanism for an unstable cervical spine injury. Stabilize his neck until you are certain there is no spine injury or other BIG 3 problem, then worry about the laceration.

Once your surveys are complete, and any more serious conditions are dealt with, you are ready to treat a soft-tissue wound. There are several steps to follow. These apply to all wounds; big and small, clean and dirty, superficial and deep, and head to toe.

Stop External Bleeding: *Direct pressure* stops most bleeding. It requires that you see clearly where the blood is coming from. You may need to cut away clothes, remove equipment, cut hair or whatever is necessary to do so. If pressure is well aimed, most bleeding stops within fifteen minutes as the clotting mechanism is activated.

If bleeding persists, it is usually because the pressure applied was too light, or was poorly aimed. Remove the bandage, find the bleeding site, and try again. Once bleeding has stopped, the clot will keep it stopped unless disturbed.

Elevation helps reduce bleeding by reducing the blood pressure in the effected extremity.

Splinting helps reduce bleeding by preventing disruption of the clot by movement.

Ice, if available, will help constrict blood vessels in the area of the injury.

Tourniquets are used ONLY with amputations—loss of a finger, hand, etc.—if severe bleeding does not stop with direct pressure. Pressure points are rarely useful in the field setting.

Prevent Infection: Long-term management (anything over two hours) requires early wound cleaning to help prevent infection. Cleansing a wound usually restarts some bleeding by disturbing the clot. If severe bleeding is a problem, leave the pressure dressing in place until bleeding is definitely stopped. *Do not attempt to clean wounds that are associated with life-threatening bleeding.*

Wash around the wound with soap and water and/or disinfectant. Clean a wide area of skin, being careful not to allow soap or disinfectant into the wound itself. The exceptions are shallow wounds, like small burns and abrasions, which can be washed with soap and water applied directly to the wound surface.

Irrigate the wound with any clean water suitable for drinking. Rinse the wound by pouring water directly into the opening and allowing water to run out by gravity. The greater the volume of water, the better. You are flushing out debris and reducing the bacteria count to levels which can be managed by the body's own defenses.

Sea water contains bacteria and can be irritating to tissues, but can be used for initial irrigation if other fresh-water sources are unavailable. Perform the final rinse with drinkable fresh water.

It is unnecessary, and can be harmful, to irrigate a wound with full strength (typically 10%) iodine preparations. Iodine kills both bacteria and body cells, leaving a partially sterilized wound lined with dead tissue. This can actually increase rather than decrease the chances of later infection. If you feel that you must use some purification, dilute the iodine to 1% by volume as an irrigation fluid.

Remove any imbedded debris from the wound. Anything which was not flushed out by irrigation should be removed manually. Brush the obvious junk out with a toothbrush or other clean tool. A pair of tweezers is useful for removing pieces of gravel or clothing that resist gentle persuasion. If a wound is very dirty, make yourself comfortable and plan to spend quite a bit of time doing this. Also remove any torn pieces of tissue in the wound that are no longer receiving blood flow. These are the pieces of skin and fat that are "hanging by a thread" or have turned blue or black.

Cover the wound with sterile dressings to prevent outside contamination. Keep the dressings as clean and dry as possible. Sterile dressing can be covered with non-sterile bandages. Re-cleanse the wound and change dressings regularly. This is usually daily, but can be more frequent in wet or dirty conditions.

Allowing the wound to drain is important. Do not close the wound with tape (butterflies or steri-strips) or try to suture it with dental floss. A closed wound has a much greater chance of getting infected than an open one. It's much easier for a surgeon to fix the scar later, if necessary, while it is healing clean and naturally.

Splint the extremity, if conditions and travel allow, if the wound is over a joint or in another area of skin which is mobile. This will minimize the breakdown of the protective barrier.

Medical Care: High-risk wounds should receive early medical attention whenever possible, especially where open fracture is suspected. Infection generally takes a day or two to get going, so your ideal evacuation plan would have your patient out of the woods within forty-eight hours. During your walk out, the wound should receive the same careful attention as any other. This is especially true for the removal of debris and irrigation. If your treatment is particularly effective, infection may never start.

Sutures (stitches) are used mainly for cosmetic purposes, to connect deep structures, and to close gaping wounds to reduce healing time. Closing a wound with sutures requires training, experience, and a scrupulously clean environment and should usually be done within 6–8 hours following the injury. In most cases, suturing is neither a necessary nor appropriate field treatment. While early suturing may be desirable for certain wounds, it can usually be safely delayed for three to five days if early treatment is not possible.

Tetanus prophylaxis is an injectable vaccine given to anyone with an open wound who has not had a vaccination within ten years, or five years in particularly dirty wounds. This is best done within twenty-four hours of injury. You can keep this from becoming a problem by keeping your routine tetanus vaccinations up to date.

Infection is a possibility in any wound, at any time during the healing process. In normal wound healing, pain, redness, and inflammation decrease with time. If the wound becomes infected, these signs and symptoms will begin to increase. Pus, an opaque white to yellow substance, may be noted in the wound and may be accompanied by a foul odor.

Almost any wound that is becoming infected earns the status of "high risk" and should receive medical care. It should continue to be treated with cleaning and dressing changes. If the infected wound has been closed with tape or sutures, it should be opened and allowed to drain. Irrigate with water to remove pus. Do not squeeze the wound, or you will just drive bacteria through the protective barrier into healthy tissues.

Warm soaks will increase circulation to the area to help the body fight the infection locally. Use only as much heat as you can comfortably stand against normal skin. Apply for thirty minutes at a time as often as five or six times a day.

Monitor for signs of infection whether or not you choose to evacuate. You should also monitor the circulation, sensation, and movement (CSM) distal to the injury as you would with a musculoskeletal problem. Bandages, splints, and swelling can create the same ischemia (lack of perfusion) here as well.

IMPALED OBJECTS

An impaled object is a foreign body that extends through the skin into underlying tissues. These are best removed by a surgeon in the hospital. If possible, stabilize impaled objects in place and transport the patient to medical care.

In many cases in the backcountry, however, transporting the patient with the object in place will cause more tissue damage than pulling it out. The impaled pick of an ice axe can do a lot of damage if the shaft bumps into a tree or rock wall. In cases such as this, removal of the object should be considered.

Remove Impaled Objects If:

1. The object prevents packaging or safe transport.

2. The object is simple, safe, and easy to remove.

ABRASIONS (Shallow Wounds)

Abrasions are shallow wounds in which only the superficial layers of skin are scraped away. Because the skin is not divided, healing can occur from the bottom up, and is usually fairly rapid. Wound-care principles are the same; stop bleeding and prevent infection.

Assessment of Abrasions: No soft tissue below the skin is visible. There is usually some ground-in dirt and there may be thin flaps of skin hanging on at the wound margins. The biggest problem with abrasions is the potential for infection. Also, you may notice that they always seem to happen in a place that's difficult to bandage.

➡ *Treatment of Abrasions:* As with lacerations, brush or pick out the foreign material, then irrigate with clean water. Any hanging and dead skin should be trimmed away. Abrasions can be covered with antibiotic ointment and dressed with sterile gauze.

Long-term care is similar to that for lacerations. Clean at least daily and redress with sterile dressing. You may use antibiotic ointment (i.e. Bacitracin, Neosporin) directly on the abrasion for pain relief and to help prevent infection. Generally, after about three or four days, the abrasion will have healed enough to allow it to dry and scab over. If this is successful, keep covered with dry dressings until it has healed completely.

BURNS

All burns are caused by heat. Damaging heat can be encountered in the form of hot gasses or objects, or be produced by a chemical reaction between the skin and caustic substance. Burns can involve internal structures, such as the Respiratory System, as well as the outside skin.

Assessment of Burns: For field management, we need to know the depth and extent of burns, as well as location. The extent is described in terms of body surface area (BSA) and is estimated using the "Rule of Nines":

Head and Neck	9%	Front of Torso	18%
Each Arm	9%	Back of Torso	18%
Each Leg	18%	Genitalia	1%

Estimates of irregular burns can be made using the size of one surface of the patient's hand, which is about 1% of the body surface area.

The depth of burn refers to how deep the damage goes. This can be difficult to estimate, particularly where different areas are burned to various degrees. To give a rough guide:

1st Degree—The skin integrity is not disrupted. Capillaries and nerves are intact. Inflammation occurs normally with redness, pain, and warmth. This is the typical sunburn.

2nd Degree—The skin surface is damaged, but the injury is limited to outer layers. Capillaries are damaged, but deeper skin blood vessels and nerves are intact, allowing inflammation to produce blisters. There is fluid loss, redness, warmth, and pain.

3rd Degree—The full thickness of skin is damaged. Capillaries, blood vessels, and nerves are destroyed. Normal inflammation cannot occur, and as a result blisters do not develop. The burned area may appear charred black, or grey. The area may not be painful due to loss of nerves. Small 3rd-degree burns may appear to be less serious because of this.

As with other injury, the assessment of burns is directed first toward identifying potentially life-threatening problems. These will usually come in the form of volume shock and/or respiratory distress. Secondary assessment considers burns which are likely to involve significant anticipated problems due to the potential for pain, infection, or scar formation. These all come under the classification of "High-Risk Burns."

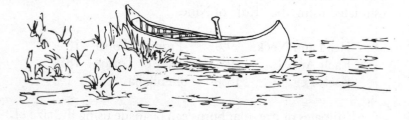

HIGH-RISK BURNS

1. *Any respiratory involvement*—Burned respiratory passages will have the same problem with inflammation, blisters, and leaking fluid that regular skin would have. Respiratory burns should be suspected in cases where the face and lips have been singed, or the patient was trapped in a closed space, such as a burning house or tent.

Respiratory distress will develop as pulmonary fluid builds up in the lungs. Swelling of the upper and lower airways can develop, producing airway constriction, and obstruction (See Respiratory System chapter). Like any other swelling, it can develop over a period of twenty-four hours. Respiratory distress should be an anticipated problem in any case where hot gasses have been inhaled, even if the patient seems to be breathing well immediately after injury.

2. *2nd- or 3rd-degree burns of the face, genitalia, hands or feet.*

3. *Burns of any degree greater than 30% BSA*—These burns have the potential to cause volume shock. The capillaries in burned skin are no longer able to contain the fluid components of the blood.

4. *3rd-degree burns greater than 10% BSA.*

5. *Chemical Burns*—It can be difficult to fully arrest the burning process as some chemicals react with the skin. Damage can continue for hours afterward.

6. *Electrical Burns*—Skin damage may be minor, but electrical current can cause extensive injury to internal organs and tissue.

7. *Burns associated with other serious injury.*

8. *Burns of very young or old patients.*

➡ **Treatment of Burns:** Stop the burning process. The first step in the management of burns is to immediately remove the heat. The fastest way to do this is immerse the patient or injured part in water. Fortunately, this is almost instinctive, as it serves to relieve pain as well. Be careful, as it is possible with larger burns to make your patient hypothermic as a side effect of your good intentions. If the burn is greater than about 10% body surface area, limit your cooling to only a few minutes.

In chemical burns, continued irrigation with water will not only cool the area, but help remove the chemical itself. Irrigation should continue for at least thirty minutes.

Treat the life-threatening injuries. If burns have the potential to cause life-threatening BIG 3 problems, use Basic Life Support techniques and request emergency evacuation.

Cleanse the burn. If the burn is not a life-threatening emergency, clean and dress it with antibiotic dressings like you would for a minor abrasion. This can be done along with the application of cool soaks for pain relief. Continue to treat as any open wound. If the burn falls under the category of "high risk," plan to have the patient to medical care as soon as possible.

BLISTERS

Mechanism of Injury: Blisters, like the kind you get on your feet while hiking, are really burns caused by the heat generated by friction. Your boots and socks rub against your skin and the damage results in leaky capillaries and swelling, and there you are. You not only have a skin injury to treat, but a transportation problem as well. Keep walking on it and you'll need a ride out of the woods just as sure as the guy with the fractured femur in the last chapter.

Assessment of Blisters: Blisters progress through three stages. They begin with "hot spots," progress to blisters filled with sterile fluid, and then break to become contaminated superficial wounds. The stage at which you confront them, and your logistical situation, will determine your treatment. Generally, they act just like other "shallow wounds."

Treatment of Blisters: Hot spots are when you begin to feel ◀ discomfort. You know something is wrong in your left boot, but you're only ten minutes into the hike you don't want to stop yet. I don't blame you, especially if the black flies are bad. But, stop you must. Outward Bound instructors, at least the smart ones, routinely stop their group early in their first hike to do a foot check and a talk on blister prevention.

Stop the friction now, and you can prevent a blister from forming. Change your socks, fiddle with your laces, or cover the sore area with smooth surface tape, gel dressings, or moleskin. You can also apply vaseline or antibiotic ointment to lubricate the area and reduce friction. Whatever time it takes to cool the hot spot will be well worth it in the long run, and save you from . . .

Blisters, which you can't always avoid. The important fact to remember early on is that a blister is a sterile wound until it breaks. Like an abrasion, the deeper layers of the skin are still intact, making quick healing from below a possibility. Whenever we can, we like to keep it that way. Small blisters can be covered with gel dressing. Larger ones will usually cause some degree of disability unless you can take the pressure off.

If the blister has formed in a bad spot, like the back of your heel, you may have to drain it in order to be able to walk. You will be converting a closed and sterile wound into an open one. We can minimize the risk of infection by treating the wound before it happens.

As with other wounds, clean the skin around and over the blister with soap and water. Sterilize a needle or sharp knife blade by flame or alcohol. Make a tiny hole in the blister at the lower margin, and allow the fluid to drain out. Leave the skin over the blister intact. It acts as its own sterile dressing. Cover the area with antibiotic ointment and dress it as you might a "hot spot." Like any open wound it must be cleaned and dressed daily and monitored for signs of infection.

Open blisters occur when a blister has broken into a non-sterile environment. It should be treated like an abrasion. Remove dead skin and debris, and cover with antibiotic ointment and sterile dressings. Remove the source of friction. Clean daily and monitor for infection.

SPARINGLY, AS OINTMENT UNDERMINES ADHESIVE FOR DRESSING.

CASE STUDY—WOUNDS

S: A six-year-old boy on Rum Cay in the Bahamian Out-Islands ran into an iron spike while playing under a pier. He had a laceration under his left eye. Other than being upset, the boy had no other complaints. He had no known allergies, and was not on medication. No one seemed to know if he had ever received tetanus immunization. The only available doctor was on Long Cay, and unable to fly over today.

O: We found an alert, cooperative, and amazingly calm six-year-old boy. There was a 3.5 centimeter laceration on the left cheek under his left eye which exposed the sub-cutaneous fat. It was contaminated with rust particles and bleeding slightly. The eye appeared to be unaffected. No bone could be seen in the wound. There was little swelling and no obvious deformity of the bones of the face. There was no neck tenderness. There was no other apparent injury. Vital Signs at 18:05 were—BP: 112/78, P: 88, R: 16, C: Alert and oriented, T: normal, Skin: normal color and temperature.

HEAD WOUND HAS POSS. MECH. FOR CERVICAL DAMAGE

A: Soft tissue wound

A': 1. Infection
     2. Tetanus

P: The bleeding was stopped with ten minutes of direct pressure. The visible pieces of rust and dirt were picked from the wound with tweezers. The area around the wound was cleaned and the wound irrigated with about two quarts of drinking water. A gauze dressing was applied. The parents were instructed to apply direct pressure if the bleeding started again and to change the dressing if it became soaked with blood. The plan was relayed to the doctor on Long Cay who was to fly over in several days. A SOAP note was left for the doctor in care of the parents.

Discussion: This was not a.wilderness scenario, but the problems were the same. I had located my own suture kit in a locker on my boat, but it had been exposed to salt water and was not fit to use. For cosmetic reasons, and to help it heal faster, the boy's wound would benefit from closure. But this did not need to happen immediately. By careful attention to cleaning the wound, we were able to preserve it for suturing several days later.

TOXINS

AND

ALLERGIES

9

TOXINS

Toxic substances can produce systemic effects, local effects, or both. Toxins, like trauma, can cause simultaneous involvement of more than one body system. The cause-and-effect relationship may be fairly obvious, or quite confusing. Treating the specific toxin requires accurate identification. The generic treatments can be applied successfully without knowing exactly what you're dealing with.

You will notice the lack of detailed drawings of various poisonous plants, insects, spiders, snakes, and other creatures. That is because specific identification is difficult, even with a color key and a lot of experience. It is also because exact identification is not the most important factor in field management. The major concern is how the body is reacting to the toxic exposure, and what you can do to lessen symptoms and prevent serious injury.

GENERAL PRINCIPLES FOR ALL TOXINS

Systemic vs. Local Effects: Systemic toxins are those which directly effect the body as a whole. They may be ingested, injected, inhaled, or absorbed through the skin. Some common examples include alcohol, mushrooms, and carbon monoxide. Local toxins affect only the immediate area of contact. These are typical of insect bites, poison ivy, and fire coral. Some toxins have both systemic and local effects. Examples are poisonous snake bite, and inhaled gasses which burn the respiratory system and are absorbed into the general circulation.

GENERAL PRINCIPLES
OF TREATMENT FOR TOXIN EXPOSURE

REMOVE AND DILUTE

Ingested Toxins: Induce vomiting. This is best done within the first hour, but may be effective up to eight hours post ingestion. Give 1–2 tablespoons (15–30 cc) syrup of Ipecac orally. Give two cups of water to dilute the toxin. The patient will vomit within twenty minutes. Be sure that the patient is positioned to prevent airway obstruction. Follow vomiting with activated charcoal (25–50 grams) mixed to a slurry with water. This will absorb and hold the remaining toxin for excretion. *Do not induce vomiting in any patient who is unable to protect their airway, or when the ingested substance is corrosive or a petroleum product.*

Inhaled Toxins: Move the patient to clean air. Provide the Generic Treatment for Respiratory Distress (See page 76).

Skin and Soft-Tissue Toxins: Clean the area as for a skin wound. Irrigate copiously with water.

General Assessment of Toxic Exposure: The signs and symptoms of specific toxins can be helpful, but are often misleading if toxins are mixed or unknown. But, it is useful to obtain as much information from the scene as possible. What was it? How much? When did it occur? If ingested plants or drugs are involved, bring samples or containers with the patient to medical care if possible.

ANTIDOTE

Effective antidotes are not always available. Certainly their use is limited in cases where the toxins are unknown or mixed. If possible, contact poison-control centers for specific treatments.

BASIC LIFE SUPPORT

Most toxins are excreted or metabolized by the body over time. Treatment is largely aimed at supporting body systems and treating problems as they develop until the toxin is removed, or can be neutralized by an antidote. This generic approach is also effective when toxins are mixed or unknown.

SPECIFIC TOXINS

—Marine Toxins, Snakebite, Insects and Arachnids

MARINE TOXINS

There are three basic mechanisms for toxic exposure in the marine environment:

1. *Spiny Injuries.* These generally produce only local effects. Examples include sting rays, scorpion fish, catfish, and some sea urchins.

2. *Nematocyst Injuries.* Nematocysts are structures in the stinging parts of jellyfish, corals, and anemones, which fire something resembling a microscopic harpoon when touched. These harpoons then inject a chemical toxin into the skin. The sensation, if you've never felt it, is like a thousand tiny bee stings. It is not a recommended vacation activity.

3. *Systemic Toxins.* The toxins of some jellyfish and a species of sea snake are known for both significant local and systemic effects. It is well worth seeking local advice about avoiding contact.

Assessment of Marine Toxins: Local effects are usually easy to identify. The pain, surprise, and indignation one feels immediately upon encountering the offending organism is usually followed by a rapid increase in the level of discomfort. The "thousands of tiny bees" sensation is typical of coral, jellyfish, and anemones. As you try to wipe away the pain you stimulate the firing of more nematocysts, and cause yourself more pain. Often jellyfish are broken up by surf and the nematocyst-bearing tentacles are floating free and almost invisible in the water. Swimming into one can be a very frightening experience because the stinging sensation continues, and you can't see what's causing it.

The sting of a poisonous ray, urchin, or fish is also obvious, and easy to distinguish from a non-toxic puncture. The pain caused by the wound itself is minimal compared to the discomfort caused by the toxin. It increases quickly with time. The barbed stinger or spine will often remain in the wound.

The systemic effects of marine toxins involve all BIG 3 systems, but respiratory distress is the most prominent symptom. Fortunately, it requires a massive exposure to most stinging marine life to have significant systemic effects.

TREATMENT OF MARINE TOXINS

Spiny Injury—The toxin is inactivated by heat. Immerse the affected part in water as hot as you can tolerate for thirty to ninety minutes or until pain is relieved. Treat the wound itself as any puncture wound. Remove the spine or stinger if possible. It will increase the chances of infection if it remains in the wound.

Nematocyst Injury—Wash off the remaining nematocysts with *salt water*, then scrap the skin in one direction, downward, with a firm-edged object like the back of your knife blade. Do not rinse in fresh water to remove nematocysts as it will stimulate them to fire. Soak or bathe the affected part in isopropyl alcohol or vinegar for thirty minutes or until pain is relieved. This will inactivate the remaining nematocysts. Powder and shave the skin to remove remaining nematocysts if pain persists.

Systemic Effects—Basic Life Support, generic wound care, and evacuation to antivenin may be wise in certain specific cases of toxic fish envenomation. Consult local authorities about the area you plan to operate in.

SNAKEBITE

In North America there are only two types of poisonous snakes to worry about, unless you happen to work in a zoo. They are pit vipers, and coral snakes. The pit vipers include rattlesnakes, copperheads, and cottonmouths. The toxin is essentially the same for all three snakes. It causes primarily local effects. The degree of systemic involvement also seen depends on the dose injected and the general health of the patient. It is interesting and useful to note that in about 40% of poisonous snake bites, venom is never injected.

Coral snake venom is primarily systemic and affects the Nervous System. It can take several hours to cause symptoms. The coral snake is a small-mouthed, shy creature. It requires some work on your part to be bitten. The victims are usually children.

Assessment of Snakebite: Identification of the snake may be helpful, but is not required for treatment. Pit vipers leave one or two fang marks. If venom has been injected (envenomation) there will be immediate swelling and pain. If no venom was injected the pain will be only what you'd expect from small puncture wounds, and won't get any worse. Be aware that Acute Stress Reaction may make this distinction difficult right after being bitten.

The fangs of the other type of poisonous snake, the coral, are quite small. The snake will have to chew its way into your skin to successfully inject venom. Its effects may be delayed for several hours. Because of this delay, the bite of a suspected coral snake must always be assumed to involve envenomation.

➡ *TREATMENT OF SNAKEBITE*

Basic Life Support
Antivenin—This is the specific treatment. Its use is usually restricted to the hospital because it can cause allergic reactions in rare cases. It is most effective during the first four hours, but can be given up to several days following the bite and still have some benefit. Pit-viper antivenin is the same for the various species of that family of snakes. It is not necessary to know the difference between a rattler, copperhead, or cottonmouth. The presence of fang marks is enough. Coral-snake antivenin, however, is specific to that species.

Transport the patient as quickly as possible to antivenin (antidote). Although local discomfort may be severe, systemic

signs and symptoms can be delayed for two to six hours following the bite. Walking your patient out is reasonably safe unless
severe systemic signs and symptoms occur. It is also significantly faster than trying a carry. Splint the affected part if
possible.

Expect Swelling—Remove constricting items such as rings,
bracelets, and clothing from the bitten extremity.

Do Not Delay—Immediately following the bite of a snake
thought to be poisonous, evacuation should be started. It can
always be slowed down or cancelled if it becomes obvious that
envenomation did not occur, or the snake was not poisonous.

   Most medical experts agree that traditional field treatments such as tourniquets, pressure dressing, ice packs, and
"cut and suck" snakebite kits are generally ineffective and are
possibly dangerous. Poisonous snakebite is one of those conditions that you cannot treat in the field. Don't waste valuable
time trying.

INSECTS AND ARACHNIDS

Insect and arachnid (spiders, scorpions) toxins are encountered
in a couple of different ways. Venom may be injected by a
stinger or specialized mouth parts as the animal attempts to de-
fend itself or warn you away from a nest. It is meant to hurt,
and it usually does. This is typical of wasps, fire ants, spiders,
and scorpions.

   More commonly, your skin reacts to the irritation of substances used by a feeding insect to prevent clotting of your
blood. Many of them also inject a local anesthetic to reduce
the pain caused by the bite, at least for as long as they're feeding. Examples of these insects include biting flies, mosquitoes,
no-see-ums, and most of the rest of the wildlife population of
North America (or so it seems).

Assessment of Insect and Arachnid Toxins: Local reaction to toxins can be severe, but involves only the extremity or immediate area of the bite or sting. There may be some degree of Acute Stress Reaction which must be distinguished from systemic effects.

Systemic Reaction: Anaphylaxis is an allergic reaction to venom or other substances. It involves the whole body with rapid, generalized swelling, hives, respiratory distress, nausea, and shock (see chapter on Anaphylaxis).

Toxin Load is the term applied to the cumulative effects of multiple stings or bites. Toxin loading can produce systemic effects which may be delayed up to twenty-four hours. This is not uncommon in blackfly country in the spring and early summer. Symptoms include fever, fatigue, headache, and nausea. This is not an allergic reaction. The generalized swelling, respiratory distress, and other signs of anaphylaxis are usually absent.

TREATMENT OF INSECT AND ARACHNID TOXINS

Local reactions are treated for comfort. Use cool soaks, elevation, and rest. Aspirin or other mild pain reliever will help. There are also a number of over-the-counter medications for insect-sting discomfort.

Systemic Reaction: Anaphylaxis is a true medical emergency. Medication, specifically epinephrine and antihistamines, can be life-saving. The indications and use of these drugs are covered in the chapter on Anaphylaxis, page 160.

Toxin Load is usually no emergency. Observe for twenty-four hours. Give aspirin or other pain reliever for comfort. Treat any problems as they develop. Keep the patient well hydrated and protected from excessive cooling or heating.

Field Treatment Summary for Toxins

Remove and Dilute
Antidote
Basic Life Support
Specific Treatments

CASE STUDY—TOXINS

S: A sixteen-year-old male on a canoe expedition in the Florida Everglades was bitten on the right arm by a four-foot snake as he was trying to throw it off his lap. The snake apparently dropped off an overhead branch. In the ensuing confusion, the snake escaped overboard. The boy was unable to describe it, other than being dark in color and very fast. He complained of pain in the mid-right forearm and feeling nauseated. The boy had no allergies and was not taking any medication. He had no past history of significant medical problems and had eaten breakfast three hours ago. There were no other recent events or injuries which could cause similar symptoms.

It was mid-morning, the sky was clear, and the temperature was about 75 degrees. The expedition was approximately seven miles from the ranger station at Flamingo.

O: The patient was Alert but pale and disoriented. He had two small puncture wounds on his right forearm. There was no swelling or discoloration. The area was tender to the touch. Distal CSM was intact. There were no other injuries. Vital Signs at 10:15 were—BP: unavailable, P: 120, R: 24, T: appears normal, Skin: pale, C: Alert but slightly disoriented.

A: 1. Snakebite—unknown if poisonous
2. Acute Stress Reaction

A': 1. Swelling and ischemia in the right arm.
2. Allergic or other systemic effects of injected toxin.

P: The right arm was splinted. The boy was placed amidships in a canoe paddled by two other people, and evacuation to the ranger station began immediately. Vital Signs and CSM checks were done every fifteen minutes. A brief SOAP note was written and sent with the patient.

Discussion: At the time of the first set of Vital Signs, the boy was found to be Alert, oriented, and relatively calm. Vital Signs were near normal. He complained of little pain of the arm. A power boat was flagged down to complete the evacuation. On arrival at the ranger station forty minutes later, the boy's condition appeared normal. It was determined that no envenomation had occurred, even though the bite was probably from a water moccasin. He was treated for puncture wounds and released, although he was advised not to return to the expedition immediately.

The evacuation of this patient was appropriate, even though it turned out that there was no emergency. Had the snake actually injected venom, the patient would have been moving in the direction of antivenin and advanced life support, had it been necessary.

— 10 —

ANAPHYLAXIS

Anaphylaxis is a severe, systemic (whole body), allergic reaction to a foreign material that enters the circulating blood. It can be caused by substances in food which are absorbed in the intestine, inhaled and absorbed through the lungs, or injected into the skin such as bee venom. The reaction to substances eaten with food may be delayed due to the time it takes to digest them. Reaction to inhaled or injected material is usually immediate (within five to fifteen minutes).

Assessment of Anaphylaxis: The signs and symptoms are caused by widespread blood-vessel dilation and tissue swelling of all body surfaces. This can produce life-threatening volume shock and airway constriction. Death can occur in a matter of minutes in severe reactions. Most patients have a history of known allergy to the suspected substance, but this is not always the case. Past reactions may have been more or less severe than the present one.

In true anaphylaxis, the patient may complain of hot, burning, itchy skin. There may be nausea, vomiting, and even diarrhea. There will be some degree of respiratory distress. The patient may feel weakness and disorientation with the onset of shock. Vital Signs are consistent with shock due to widespread blood-vessel dilation and respiratory distress due to lower airway constriction (see Circulatory System, Respiratory System).

Vital Signs in Anaphylaxis

P: increased
R: increased with distress / wheezing if severe
BP: decreased if severe
C: anxious / confused; V, P, or U if severe
S: flushed with hives, general swelling
T: unchanged

Survey will reveal generalized swelling of the face, eyes, tongue, and skin. Do not confuse anaphylaxis with a severe *local* reaction, such as a swollen arm after a bee sting. The anaphylaxis patient will almost always have altered mental status, and may not be responsive. It is easy to mistake anaphylaxis for seizure or Acute Stress Reaction. Assessment can be difficult if there is no history to go on.

➡️ **Treatment of Anaphylaxis:** Provide Basic Life Support as you would for any patient with shock and respiratory distress. However, specific treatment with drugs is generally required to reverse severe reactions. This works best if done in the field, before the reaction has progressed to a critical condition.

The drug most frequently used is injectable Epinephrine, which is the synthetic version of the hormone adrenalin. It reverses the effects of severe reactions by causing systemic constriction of blood vessels. The drug is supplied specifically for this purpose in the form of "Bee-Sting Kits" which contain a pre-loaded and calibrated hypodermic syringe. They are available at any pharmacy by prescription from your doctor. It is strongly recommended that you or anyone in your group who has a known insect allergy obtain and carry one of these kits and be familiar with its use.

Be aware that epinephrine does not remove or neutralize the foreign material which caused the reaction. It is possible to see a "rebound reaction" with reappearance of symptoms minutes or hours later when the epinephrine wears off. Multiple doses may be necessary.

Antihistamines are also used in the treatment of anaphylaxis. These drugs do not reverse blood vessel dilation or vascular shock, but can help prevent further reaction to histamine and rebound effect. Any antihistamine is helpful, even the stuff in your over-the-counter cold medication. Benadryl (diphenhydramine) is the most common.

Since the effects of epinephrine are temporary, evacuation should be instituted at once. If the patient has recovered from the event, it need not be an emergency. Careful monitoring for rebound reaction is crucial. Also, be aware that a second exposure to the same foreign material can cause an even more severe reaction.

SECTION V

ENVIRONMENTAL MEDICINE

11

PROBLEMS WITH
BODY-CORE TEMPERATURE

The core of the human body operates most efficiently at or very near a temperature of 98.6 degrees F (37.2 centigrade). Even a small change in either direction can adversely affect the normal chemical reactions that are part of all body processes. Fortunately, a healthy body can control its internal temperature by balancing heat loss and heat production against the challenges of environmental conditions.

You are usually a willing participant. You put on or shed clothing, seek the shade when you're hot, or lie in sun like a lizard when you're cold. You curl up to preserve heat, or spread yourself out to get rid of it. Your intelligence and freedom of movement are two of the factors used in striking the balance.

Much of the process is unconscious. You don't have to

think about it. The body's compensatory mechanisms constrict blood vessels in the skin to keep heat in the core, or dilate them to radiate excess heat. Sweat glands release fluid to enhance cooling by evaporation. Shivering is the body's attempt to produce heat by involuntary exercise. While you can watch them work, these mechanisms are not under your direct control.

Problems with temperature regulation develop when the compensatory mechanisms fail, due to injury, illness, accident, or ignorance. As you should have guessed, one of the first signs of abnormal core temperature is a change in consciousness and mental status (C). You rapidly lose your judgment and common sense, and from there, the problems only get worse.

Hyperthermia and hypothermia are systemic problems involving too much heat, or too little heat, in the body core. With each we can define three distinct stages. The first stage is the body's normal and healthy response to the environmental challenge. The second marks the failure of the compensatory mechanisms and mild changes in core temperature. The third stage represents a severe, life-threatening condition with complete loss of temperature regulation.

SEVERE HYPOTHERMIA	MILD HYPOTHERMIA	COLD RESPONSE	NORMAL	HEAT RESPONSE	HEAT EXHAUSTION	HEAT STROKE
DESPERATE PROBLEM	URGENT PROBLEM		RANGE OF NORMAL FUNCTION		URGENT PROBLEM	DESPERATE PROBLEM

*Avoiding problems with body-core temperature
requires keeping yourself within the range
of normal function.*

HYPERTHERMIA (ELEVATED BODY TEMPERATURE)

Heat Challenge vs. Passive Heat Loss + Active Heat Loss:
Factors in the heat challenge are both internal and external. The internal contribution is the body's production of heat

through metabolism and exercise. The external factors include the temperature of the surrounding environment, air movement (wind), and humidity.

The body attempts to balance these effects by passive and active heat-loss mechanisms. Passive heat loss relies on the ability of the body to radiate heat. Skin blood vessels can be dilated to bring heat to the surface where it can be lost to the environment. We consciously assist this mechanism by removing insulating clothing and spreading our extremities to the wind.

Active heat loss is accomplished by sweating. Water absorbs heat from the skin as it evaporates, so the body constantly sacrifices fluid to maintain normal temperature in hot environments. The effectiveness of sweating is limited by the volume of fluid available to produce sweat.

Water will evaporate very quickly into air that is dry, and slowly or not at all into air that is already saturated with water. Sweating is a much more efficient method of heat loss in very dry environments. In fact, sweat can evaporate so quickly in dry climates that profuse sweating may go unnoticed until fluid loss is severe. In high humidity the amount of fluid lost to sweat will be much more obvious as it runs into your eyes and drips off your nose because it can't evaporate. The low rate of evaporation also prevents efficient cooling.

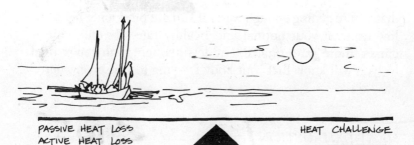

PASSIVE HEAT LOSS
ACTIVE HEAT LOSS   HEAT CHALLENGE

Maintaining normal function means retaining
a balance between body temperature
and the elements.

HEAT RESPONSE

Here we see the body's passive and active heat-loss mechanisms at work. The blood vessels in the body shell (skin) are dilated, and sweat is being produced. Fluid is being sacrificed at a prodigious rate.

Assessment of Heat Response: The mechanisms for shedding heat are working, and the body temperature is near-normal. Level of consciousness and mental status are still normal. The person (note: not yet a patient) is responding appropriately to the heat challenge by reducing exercise, removing clothing, seeking shade, replacing fluid, and so on, as needed to maintain normal body temperature. Common sense is intact.

➡ *Treatment of Heat Response:* No specific treatment is required. Common sense should tell you that keeping the balance between heat challenge and heat loss is critical. Pushing yourself or others out of balance is asking for trouble. When the signs of heat response are present, pay attention to fluid replacement, maximizing heat losses, and minimizing heat challenge.

While you're thinking about this, it is important to point out that being thirsty is a relatively late sign of fluid depletion. By the time you feel thirst, your tank is already getting low. In the face of Heat Challenge, drink before you become thirsty!

A better sign of fluid status is urine output. You'll know that you're getting enough water if you are producing light yellow urine at your normal and healthy rate. If your urine is darker (more concentrated) and less frequent than you're used to, you will know that your body is trying to conserve water.

HEAT EXHAUSTION   *p. 55*   <105°

This is the beginning of trouble. Heat exhaustion is really early volume shock caused by dehydration (sweating losses exceeding fluid intake). The term is a little misleading, however, because core temperature is not yet significantly elevated.

Assessment of Heat Exhaustion: You will recognize the vital sign pattern as mild compensated volume shock (see Chapter 4) including the shell/core effect. In the backcountry, heat exhaustion is a serious problem which requires immediate treatment.

Vital Signs in Heat Exhaustion

    BP: normal or decreased
     P: increased
     R: increased
     S: variable, may be flushed or clammy and
         sweaty
     T: normal or slightly elevated (below 105°)
   *C: usually Alert with normal mental status

    Urine Output is decreased, as the body seeks to preserve fluid balance.
    General Condition will be weak, thirsty, and nauseated. Vomiting is common.

Treatment of Heat Exhaustion: Reduce the heat challenge by moving the patient into the shade. Stop physical exertion, fan the patient with air, and assist evaporative cooling with water. The object is to stop the progression of volume shock by stopping fluid loss through sweating. Radical cooling, such as immersion in ice water, is not necessary.
    Fluid replacement should begin immediately. Oral intake is usually adequate, but intravenous fluid is faster if available. Oral replacement is still possible even if the patient is vomiting by giving fluid frequently in small amounts. Look for urine production as an indication of the return of normal fluid volume.

Replacing salt is a good idea following heavy sweating, but is not necessary for emergency treatment. Salt, if you're worried about it, is provided by most foods. Do not use salt tablets, which cause stomach irritation and vomiting.

HEAT STROKE

This is a true medical emergency. The active and passive heat-loss mechanisms are overwhelmed by the heat challenge and the body's core temperature rises out of control to critical levels (greater than 105°). The patient's fluid volume status depends on the rate of rise in temperature. Contrary to what is described in some first-aid texts. It *is* possible to have heat stroke and still be sweating.

In a state of fluid depletion, heat exhaustion results in loss of effective sweating (sweating absent) and precedes a rise in core temperature. This could occur after hiking all day in a warm environment with limited water intake. In the presence of an extreme heat challenge a critical rise in core temperature can occur before fluid stores are depleted (sweating still present). This can be caused by forced exercise in a hot environment. It can also be caused by staying in the sauna too long.

Assessment of Heat Stroke: Regardless of how quick the onset, these people are very sick. There are unmistakable changes in Level of Consciousness. Severe mental status changes will rapidly lead to a drop on the AVPU scale. The skin may have the classic hot, red, and dry appearance, but this is not a reliable sign. If the fluid volume is intact it may be wet with sweat, or clammy due to shock. The key indicators are a positive mechanism for hyperthermia, a high core temperature, and any changes in Level of Consciousness.

Vital Signs in Heat Stroke

BP: Variable to decreased
P: Increased

R: Increased
S: Variable, may be flushed or clammy, may be dry
or sweaty
T: Severely elevated above 105°F
*****C:**   Changes in Consciousness preceded by MS
changes (hallucinating, agitated, etc.). May also
have seizures.

Treatment of Heat Stroke: This is a life-threatening emergency requiring immediate field treatment. There is no time for delay. Once hyperthermia has reached this point, the chances of survival are not good.

Radical cooling is required. The best method is immediate immersion in cold water. If this method is used, you must monitor core temperature to prevent hypothermia. If no thermometer is available, look for an improvement in Consciousness and mental status to determine the return of more normal temperature. If no pond, river, or ocean is available, pour whatever water you have onto the skin and fan vigorously.

Fluid replacement is critical. Normal cooling requires normal volume. Oral fluid replacement is too slow and is impossible in the unresponsive patient. Intravenous replacement is clearly the treatment of choice, but not in everybody's backpack.

Basic Life Support is instituted to preserve vital functions while cooling. The recovery of a heat-stroke patient is dependent on quick, radical field treatment. It is rarely a problem that makes it to the hospital.

Evacuation is necessary even if you succeed in reducing the core temperature in time to save the patient. These people have suffered a severe injury and require treatment and observation in the hospital. Brain injury and/or shock are common. Emergency evacuation is certainly justified.

Field Treatment Summary for Hyperthermia

Heat Response—Maintain Balance: replace fluids, reduce exercise, increase heat loss.

Heat Exhaustion—Immediately Reduce Heat Challenge, Replace Fluid Volume.

Heat Stroke—Radical Cooling

HYPOTHERMIA (REDUCED BODY TEMPERATURE)

Cold Challenge* vs. *Heat Retention* + *Heat Production:
Our good friend and colleague, John Haskins, is a superb Outward Bound instructor. He's had a lot of first-hand experience with hypothermia. John has spent too much time in small, open boats off the coast of Maine. No one could design a better laboratory for studying the effects of long-term exposure to cold and wet environments. Like hyperthermia, one of the first things to be affected by hypothermia is judgment and common sense. The fact that he keeps going back out there seems to prove this point.

The Maine Coast is particularly good at providing all the elements of the Cold Challenge; a low ambient temperature, wetness in the form of rain, fog, and general high humidity, and wind. To counter the challenge, John uses passive heat retention in the form of insulation (fat and winter clothing), and constriction of the blood vessels in the skin to keep warmth in the core (shell/core effect). He also reduces the area of his body exposed to heat loss by curling up in the bottom of the boat. By this time John is usually cold, shivering, and miserable.

He is quick to recognize the shell/core effect and his body's attempt to produce heat, he leaps to an oar and rows briskly to help with active heat production. His students think he's crazy, but John is beginning to feel better. He also knows that in order to produce heat, he needs calories to burn. This is a perfect excuse to eat something. Now John feels much better. He may still be at sea, lost in the fog, but at least he's warm.

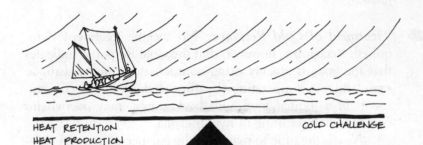

HEAT RETENTION
HEAT PRODUCTION   COLD CHALLENGE

COLD RESPONSE

Here are the body's heat-retention and heat-production mechanisms at work. The shell/core effect reduces blood flow to the skin, reducing heat loss to the environment. There may be shivering as the body attempts to produce heat from muscular exercise.

Another interesting phenomenon associated with the Cold Response is "cold diuresis." This is the tendency of the body to produce more urine when shell/core compensation occurs. Fluid depletion can be a problem in hypothermia as well as hyperthermia, but in this case urine output becomes a problem rather than an indicator of good fluid volume.

Assessment of Cold Response: Since the compensation mechanisms are working, the core temperature is normal. Level of Consciousness and Mental Status are normal. The skin will be pale and cool with the person (not yet a patient) feeling uncomfortably cold. Shivering may be slight, or very obvious.

➡ *Treatment of Cold Response:* No specific treatment is required. Recognize, however, that the Cold Response indicates that the body is already using compensatory mechanisms to maintain core temperature. Further changes in the environment, or a limited food and fluid supply, may overwhelm compensation resulting in hypothermia.

Now is the time to maintain the balance of thermal regulation by reducing the cold challenge and increasing heat retention and production. Beware of trying to produce heat without calories to burn. *Living outside in a cold environment can require more than 6000 calories a day. This is no time to be on a diet, and no time to be lying passively in cold bilge water. Get into dry clothing, eat, and exercise.*

Cold diuresis, and the logistics involved in obtaining fresh water in an extreme environment, can lead to fluid volume depletion. Normal volume is necessary for normal heat production. Make the additional effort to keep yourself well hydrated.

The onset of hypothermia is insidious more often than dramatic. Any idiot can diagnose hypothermia in someone who's been overboard in The Gulf of Maine for twenty minutes. The usual case, however, creeps up on you because you allow yourself or someone else to be just a little cold for a long time. Awareness of the potential for the problem must be coupled with action to prevent it *before* your common sense and judgment are affected.

WARM INSULATED TRAIL DRINKS

MILD HYPOTHERMIA

in.PA · SEZ
90 - 96°

Passive heat retention and active heat production are overwhelmed by the Cold Challenge and the body-core temperature falls below 95 degrees fahrenheit. This can occur rapidly, as in cold-water immersion, or slowly over hours or days. Hypothermia can often co-exist with other problems. It can be a complication of trauma, intoxication, altitude sickness, or any other condition which reduces a person's resistance to the cold challenge.

Hypothermia can contribute to injury or death from other mechanisms. Most drowning, for example, occurs because the extremities become uncoordinated as the body shell cools by exposure to cold water. Hypothermia can lead to errors in judgment resulting in falls while rock climbing, or working on a slippery deck offshore. It must always be suspected in any problem occurring in a cool setting.

Assessment of Mild Hypothermia: In rapid onset cases (overboard in the Gulf of Maine for twenty minutes), the body's fuel stores of available calories have not been used up. There is often a radical difference in temperature between the body shell (skin), and the body core. In slow onset cases, fuel stores are often depleted. The temperature difference between shell and core is not as dramatic. The gradual appearance of symptoms may be difficult for the patient and rescuer to recognize.

The most obvious outward signs of mild hypothermia are mild to moderate mental status changes and shivering. The patient may be lethargic and withdrawn, irritable, and lose problem-solving ability and judgment. The skin will be pale and cool, and there may be some loss of dexterity in extremities as the shell/core effect reduces blood flow. Shivering can be mild to severe as the body forces muscles to exercise to generate heat. If fluid volume is not already depleted, cold diuresis will continue with the patient producing relatively dilute urine.

↓ "WHEN LAST URINATED?" ; COLOR? AMT?

↓ (FLUID DEPLETED YET OR NOT?)

Vital Signs in Mild Hypothermia

P: Normal
BP: Normal
R: Normal
T: 90–96 degrees F   vs 98.6° ± 1°
*C: A on AVPU, Mild to moderate MS changes
S: Shell/core effect

Temperatures are best measured rectally, if possible. Shell cooling will cause oral readings to be lower than the core temperature. A special low-reading clinical thermometer is required for measuring core temperature below 94 degrees F.

➡ **Treatment of Mild Hypothermia:** Mild hypothermia is an urgent field problem. Unless positive changes occur in the temperature of the outside environment, the body's heat retention, or the body's heat production, severe hypothermia will soon follow. Field rewarming must be an immediate priority to prevent further problems. Any field-rewarming technique is generally safe. The several options available allow you to choose a procedure to fit the conditions.

1. *Reduce the Cold Challenge*—Reduce the Cold Challenge by sheltering the patient from the wind and wet. Remove wet and cold clothing. Add heat to the environment. Build a fire, lay the patient in the sun, or surround him with warm bodies. The addition of heat to insulating materials helps prevent further cooling, but does not generally cause significant rewarming. Avoid placing anything hot directly on the skin, as the patient may not be able to feel a developing burn.

2. *Heat Rentention*—Clothe or wrap the patient in dry insulation with special attention to the head and face. A vapor barrier over your insulation, like a plastic or a foil blanket, will reduce evaporative cooling and the effect of wind and aid in heat retention. Be sure to insulate from the cold ground as well.

3. *Heat Production*—Produce body heat by providing quick calories, fluids, and exercise. The fastest way to make calories available for heat production is to feed the patient foods containing lots of simple sugars. This means Twinkies, candy bars, and hot chocolate. This simple energy will be absorbed quickly and burn fast, which is exactly what is needed right now.

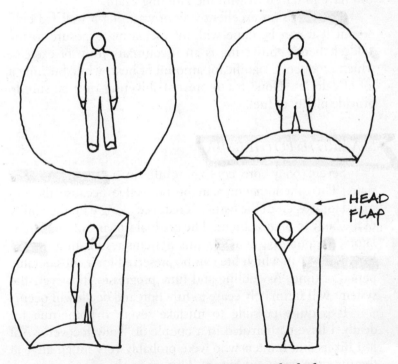

HEAD FLAP

The human burrito. This wrap method of insulating allows quick and easy access to the patient, as well as protection.

Once the patient has warmed up a bit, and his digestive systems is working again, fuel stores can be replenished with more complex carbohydrates, fats, and proteins. Now is the time for warmer and less desperate trailside dining with your tofu, whole-grain pancakes, and bacon, which will provide a more steady and long-lasting source of energy. Either that, or send out for a pizza.

This is really just the same concept that you use to start a campfire. First comes the birch bark and kindling which lights with a match and burns like crazy. Once the heat is available, you add the sticks and logs. If you're successful, you have a nice, even-burning, night-long source of heat. Let it die, and you have to start over with the kindling again.

Exercise is an excellent way of warming a well fed cold person if it can be done without increasing exposure to the cold challenge. Shivering is an involuntary form of exercise which produces a significant amount of heat, while burning a lot of calories. Don't try to prevent shivering, just be sure to provide plenty of fuel.

SEVERE HYPOTHERMIA

Severe body-core cooling results in a hibernation-like state. This phenomenon can be protective because the demand for oxygen in the tissues is reduced along with the ability of the body to perfuse them. The gradual slowing of the Circulatory, Respiratory, and Nervous Systems results in a "metabolic icebox" in which life can be preserved for a considerable period of time. As cooling and time progresses, however, the systems will ultimately cease to function and death will occur.

It is quite possible to mistake severe hypothermia for death. I have participated in a couple of "body recoveries" of lost hikers and hunters who were probably very much alive at the time the carry-out began. This was only a few years ago, but no one knew much about the metabolic icebox. Fortunately, recent advances in the understanding and treatment of severe hypothermia have resulted in completely different field management, and the survival of patients who would have otherwise been given up for dead.

Assessment of Severe Hypothermia: The distinction between mild and severe hypothermia is critically important for field treatment. Accurate measurement of core temperature by rectal thermometer can be very helpful when you're trying to decide how to treat.

As the core temperature falls below 90 degrees F, mental status changes will be severe, leading to a decrease in level of consciousness. The severe hypothermic may exhibit bizarre personality changes, hallucinations, and confusion, followed by a drop to V, P, or U on the AVPU scale. This is quite different from the lethargic but responsive mild hypothermic. Shivering will *stop* as shell cooling and lack of calories to burn deactivates muscles. Cold diuresis may continue if fluid stores are not yet depleted.

Vital Signs in Severe Hypothermia

P: Decreased. May be as slow as one beat per minute.
BP: Decreased. May be unobtainable.
R: Decreased. May not be observable.
T: Below 90 degrees F.
*C: Severe MS changes leading to decreased level of consciousness.
S: Cold, pale.

Treatment of Severe Hypothermia: Field rewarming can be dangerous and is usually ineffective. Severely hypothermic patients should be transported as quickly as possible to controlled rewarming in a hospital. The "metabolic icebox" effect is protective, but only for a limited time. During evacuation, the following steps should be taken as the situation allows:

Transport gently because cold heart muscle is extremely irritable. Jostling or other rough handling can cause ventricular fibrillation. Do not exercise the patient. Ventilation may be performed if respiration is deemed inadequate.

Position the patient flat. The blood vessels in the body shell have lost their ability to constrict and will allow blood to escape the core if the patient is held upright. If the patient must be lowered down a cliff, or hoisted into a helicopter, do it only with the patient positioned horizontally in a litter.

Apply mild heat only. External heat sources such as heat packs help prevent further heat loss and can be safely used. However, active rewarming, such as a hot bath, is difficult to control and dangerous.

Package the patient in dry insulation, such as a sleeping bag, and a vapor barrier, such as a tent fly or ground cloth, to prevent further heat loss.

Field Treatment Summary for Hypothermia

Cold Response—Maintain balance between Cold Challenge and Heat Production and Retention: eat, drink, exercise, insulate.

Mild Hypothermia—Field Rewarming

Severe Hypothermia—Evacuate to Controlled Rewarming

CASE STUDY—HYPOTHERMIA

S: A 17-year-old male student was removed from the bow of a pulling boat after being on watch without relief for three hours during a cold and wet sail to windward. He had repeatedly been asked if he was cold, or would like something to eat, and always has replied "OK." He responded the same way when asked if he saw anything ahead. Since no one else was particularly excited about replacing him, he remained at his post. Eventually, someone noticed that his wool hat had rolled down over his eyes even though he continued to claim to be on lookout. After some debate among the students, this was brought to the instructor's attention.

The student had no known allergies, he was not on medication, he had no history of significant medical problems, and his last meal was over four hours before. There was no reason to suspect trauma.

O: On examination, the student was lethargic but responsive to verbal stimuli. He could open his eyes and sit up on command. His foul-weather gear was open in front and he was soaked to the waist. Vital Signs at 16:15 were—BP: 110/70, P: 60, R: 12, C: V on AVPU, T: felt cool, Skin: pale.

A: Mild Hypothermia

A': Severe Hypothermia

P: Sail was reduced and the boat was turned downwind. One student was detailed to start the stove, and another to replace the patient on watch. Other students removed the patient's soaked gear. He was clothed in borrowed polypropylene, placed in a doubled sleeping bag, and wrapped in a plastic tarp. He was assisted in drinking a couple of cups of warm, thick cocoa.

Discussion: Although this problem could have been avoided, it was handled appropriately once discovered. The instructor's plan stabilized the scene, reduced the cold challenge and increased heat retention and production.

This fellow showed almost immediate improvement in Level of Consciousness and mental status. Evacuation was not initiated, but the instructor chose to continue downwind to an anchorage several miles away. The expedition was continued in the same messy and cold easterly wind the following day, but the entire crew was warm, well fed, and hydrated.

12

COLD INJURY

Exposure to temperatures below 32 degrees F can freeze body tissues. Any factors which reduce the circulation of warm blood to tissues allow freezing to occur more readily. In people who are already a little chilled, the cold response with "shell/ core effect" reduces perfusion to the extremities to maintain core temperature. Constricting clothing, such as ski boots or a splint tied too tight, can reduce blood flow as well. Cigarette smoking can be an additional factor, infusing the body tissues with nicotine, which is a powerful vasoconstrictor.

I will forever be amazed by the sight of a lightly dressed skier huddled on the chairlift with the temperature below zero, having his morning cigarette. He should just take off all his clothes, jump in the snow, and get it over with! Few of them seem to see what skiing hatless and smoking has to do with frostbitten toes. The ski boots are usually blamed.

This is not such a big deal at a ski resort with lodges top and bottom. But in the backcountry, dealing with frostbite is inconvenient at best, and often disastrous. It must be taken seriously, both in prevention and in cure.

Certainly, well insulated and fitted boots, gloves, and a face mask can go a long way toward preventing frostbite in extreme conditions. But equally important is maintaining an active and warm body core. This will ensure a good supply of warm blood to the extremities. That's why you eat a good breakfast and wear a hat to keep your feet warm.

Sometime when you're not paying attention, or you are a little hypothermic and not thinking clearly enough to prevent it, tissues will begin to freeze. You won't feel it happening. Remember that nerve tissue is the most sensitive to oxygen deprivation, so when circulation stops, the affected part goes numb. Ice crystals form, doing the same kind of damage ice can do anywhere. The same forces that can crack the granite cliffs you are climbing are at work damaging the cells in your skin and soft tissues.

The very early stage of freezing is called "frostnip." This occurs when there is a loss of local tissue perfusion with the beginning of ice-crystal formation. Only the outer layers of skin are affected and damage is minimal. Prompt rewarming at this stage usually causes no disability or tissue loss.

Severe damage can result with prolonged or very deep freezing. Much of the damage occurs during and after rewarming. Rewarmed tissue is very sensitive to further injury, even from normal use, and refreezing is devastating.

Assessment of Cold Injury

Frostnip is the loss of circulation due to early freezing of the superficial layers of the skin. The area will appear white or grey (pink or red in dark-skinned people) and feel cold and stiff to the touch. However, the area will remain pliable enough to allow movement over unfrozen deeper layers, joints, and tendons. The typical discomfort of early cooling will be replaced by numbness.

Frostnip responds rapidly to rewarming. There will be pain during treatment, with only mild inflammation following. The rewarmed skin will be mildly tender, red, and slightly swollen. Blistering generally does not occur. No specific long-term care is required, although the skin will be more susceptible to further cold injury.

Frostbite occurs when the skin and underlying tissues are frozen solid. The area is white or bluish and firm to touch. Skin does not move over joints or underlying tissues. Ice crystals are usually visible on the skin surface. There is a complete loss of sensation. The digit or extremity feels like a club.

Rewarming is extremely painful and can cause further damage if not done properly. The rewarmed tissues do not look or feel normal. There will be signs of mild to severe inflammation with blisters, swelling, and redness. There may be some death of tissue which will appear dark blue or black.

Treatment of Cold Injury: *Frostnip* should be immediately rewarmed at the first sign of numbness. Left frozen, frostnip can easily progress to frostbite. Like early hypothermia, frostnip is a case for stopping whatever you're doing and making the time and effort to warm up. Any method which does not cause tissue damage is fine. Usually just sheltering or covering the area better will do it. Remember to warm the whole body as well as the affected part. Reverse the shell/core effect. Put a hat on, eat something, and exercise to produce heat. The people who get into trouble with frostbite are the ones who ignore the first signs of frostnip.

Frostbite is best treated by rewarming under controlled conditions. The chances of further damage from trauma and infection are high. Pain will be severe. Usually this means the patient should be in a hospital. Keeping tissue in the frozen state for several hours during an evacuation is generally a better plan than uncontrolled field rewarming. This is especially true of frozen feet and hands, which will be impossible to use once rewarmed.

Occasionally deep frostbite rewarms spontaneously as the

shell/core effect is reversed by exercise or insulation during the walk out. There is no way to safely prevent this rewarming (do not pack frozen extremities in snow, for example). It is vital to prevent trauma to the rewarmed part. This generally means no use of the digit or extremity. Absolutely never allow the part to refreeze. Consider rewarmed frostbite to be a high-risk wound. Bandages and splinting are required. If we're talking about rewarmed frostbitten feet, a carry-out evacuation is required.

Be sure to keep the patient warm, dry, well fed, and hydrated. Monitor distal circulation, sensation, and movement frequently to ensure that splints or bandages do not constrict circulation as swelling develops. If possible, keep the part elevated. Early medical follow-up is essential.

TRENCH FOOT

Trench foot is an injury that develops with prolonged exposure to cold and wet conditions above freezing. It is not limited to feet, and often involves the hands as well. Numbness is common, for example, in hands of river paddlers on a cold day. This numbness is due to decreased circulation (perfusion) only and does not indicate frost bite. However, tissue damage can occur if the conditions persist over days or weeks.

The same conditions can be duplicated by wearing vapor-barrier boots in cold conditions. High-altitude climbers, and sailors or fishermen at sea in circumstances which do not permit adequate drying, are a set-up for trench foot.

Assessment of Trench Foot: The history is usually the key. The signs and symptoms are typical of a general inflammatory response with pain, redness, and sometimes blisters. If not adequately treated, secondary infection can develop.

➡ *Treatment of Trench Foot (or hand):* If the cause is wet and cold, the treatment must be warm and dry. Like frostbite, healing tissue can be damaged by further use. Bandaging may be required. Treat as you would any other soft-tissue injury, to prevent infection and allow healing.

Prevention is worth the trouble. In "trench" conditions, try to give your hands and feet several dry and warm hours each day. Sleep with your wet socks in your sleeping bag to dry, but not on your feet. Take your wetsuit booties and gloves off whenever possible. Inside vapor-barrier boots, change socks frequently to keep your feet as dry as you can. (Related material: chapter on Skin and Soft Tissue.)

Field Treatment for Cold Injury

Extremity Cooling—Reverse Shell/Core Effect: eat, exercise, drink, insulate.

Frost Nip—Immediate Field Rewarming

Frost Bite—Evacuate to Controlled Rewarming: protect any rewarmed parts from trauma and re-freezing

Trench Foot—Dry and Warm

13

NEAR DROWNING

Drowning refers to death by respiratory failure because liquid gets in the way of gas exchange in the lung. The liquid is usually water, and it usually comes from outside the body. This generally occurs when the patient inhales part of the lake, ocean, or river in which he or she is submerged.

The most common cause of drowning is loss of muscular coordination due to the rapid shell cooling that occurs in cold-water immersion. No longer able to swim, the patient sinks below the surface and inhales water. Even the strongest swimmer can drown this way.

Drowning can also happen almost instantly with the involuntary gasp that sometimes comes with the surprise of sudden immersion. This can affect kayakers rolled by a wave, or fisherman pulled out of the boat by their pot warp or nets.

They are immediately deprived of any reserve air and will not remain conscious for more than a few seconds. Most of the time, water fills the lungs all the way to the alveoli. In about 15% of the cases, the larynx goes into spasm, closing off the lungs and resulting in a "dry drowning."

In either case, a water-filled respiratory system is unhealthy, but not always fatal. The term "near-drowning" indicates at least temporary survival of water inhalation. This occurs in very cold water where the rapid onset of hypothermia offers temporary protection to the brain deprived of oxygen. In rare cases in the civilized setting, patients have been resuscitated after up to an hour under cold water with little or no long-term brain damage. What is meant by "cold" is controversial. Generally, though, any water below about 70 degrees F can be considered cold enough to have the desired effect. The degree of protection offered by the onset of hypothermia probably increases considerably as water temperature goes down.

Assessment of Near Drowning: This is a Primary Survey problem. You are looking at the Airway, Breathing, Circulation, and Disability. Evaluation includes determining how long the patient was submerged, how cold the water is, and how soon advanced life support can be reached. Resuscitation should be attempted if the patient has been in the water for less than an hour.

Treatment of Near Drowning: Respiratory failure is a BIG 3 problem, and is treated immediately with artificial ventilation. There is no need to drain water from the lungs, and there is no difference in field treatment between salt and fresh water. Confirmed pulselessness (cardiac arrest) is treated with chest compressions.

When hypothermia is a factor, the pulse can be very difficult to find. While continuing ventilations, be very thorough in determining the absence of a pulse before beginning chest compressions; this may take as long as two minutes but it re-

duces the chance of damaging a functioning heart that has
been slowed by hypothermia.

Most of the people who survive drowning *have* functional
heart activity, and respond to ventilation within the first two
minutes while you are still feeling for a pulse. These people
have suffered a serious injury and are still at risk for respiratory
distress. Water is an irritant to lung tissue, and will cause the
later development of pulmonary edema (fluid in the lungs).
Even though they may appear to be recovering, they should be
quickly evacuated to medical care.

Those who are in cardiac arrest when they are pulled
from the water have a much lower survival rate. In the urban
setting, Basic Life Support with Cardio-Pulmonary Resuscitation begins immediately. Rapid transport to a hospital with
well controlled resuscitation and rewarming follows close behind. There have been a few dramatic resuscitations performed this way.

In the wilderness environment, success with patients who
do not respond quickly to Basic Life Support is less likely. The
question of further treatment is controversial. Some authorities suggest that these patients should be treated as severe hypo-
thermics, packaged to prevent heat loss, and transported gently
to controlled rewarming in a hospital.

14

ACUTE MOUNTAIN SICKNESS (ALTITUDE SICKNESS)

An increase in altitude by foot, car, plane, or hot-air balloon changes the atmospheric environment around you. The higher you go, the less oxygen there is. At about 18,000 feet above sea level, air pressure is reduced by 50%. This is accentuated at higher latitudes because the earth's atmosphere is thicker at the equator and thinner at the poles. Thus, the effects of altitude on the summit of Denali in Alaska are about 15% greater than at the same altitude in the Himalayas.

At a constant altitude, the amount of oxygen in the air is constant. It does not fluctuate significantly with the temperature, time of day, season, or any other routine environmental changes. Your BIG 3 body systems become accustomed to this. Your rate of respiration, the number of red blood cells in your circulation, and other physiologic parameters are in balance with your environment, whether you're a lobsterman or a mountain guide.

There are compensatory mechanisms which allow you to change altitude, within limits, without getting out of balance. You can move from sea level to about 8000 feet with minimal effect. In the short term, there will be an increase in respiratory rate with associated chemical changes (elevated pH) in the blood. If you stay several days, your kidneys will re-balance the pH of the blood, resetting your system to your new environment.

If you were to continue even higher, your body would compensate and re-balance again. Over the course of weeks, you would undergo further physiologic changes, like producing more red blood cells. Ultimately, you would reach the limit of your body's ability to compensate.

This ability of your body to adapt to altitude, and the speed with which it happens, varies widely from person to person. It appears to have no relationship to physical fitness or gender. Some people adapt to altitude better than others. However, everyone's ability to adapt to higher altitudes is reduced by dehydration, alcohol and depressant drugs, and overexertion.

The best way to adapt to higher altitude is to take your time, maintain hydration, stay away from depressants, and take it easy. Allow your normal compensatory mechanisms the time necessary to work by ascending in stages. Climb no faster than your body can adapt. Do not overexert on the first day at the new altitude, and plan to remain for two to three days before proceeding higher. If you pay attention to what your body is trying to tell you, you should be able to avoid the more severe forms of altitude sickness.

Severe altitude sickness develops when the reduced oxygen availability results in capillary leakage and generalized body-tissue swelling. The organs most seriously affected by this are the brain and lungs, producing the symptoms of the medical problem we call Acute Mountain Sickness (AMS). These two major components are called High Altitude Pulmonary Edema (HAPE), and High Altitude Cerebral Edema (HACE).

Assessment of AMS: In the early stages, symptoms are attributable to the chemical effects of having less oxygen per breath, and the work the body has to do to make up for it. Later, more serious symptoms appear as edema develops throughout the body. Its effects are first noticed in the lungs and brain. Severe altitude sickness includes the effects of pulmonary fluid and increased intracranial pressure (see chapters 5 and 6).

Mild AMS is characterized by mild headache easily relieved by aspirin or ibuprofen and slight nausea with little or no vomiting. The patient may experience slight dizziness, loss of appetite, and mild fatigue. There is usually some degree of insomnia and increased shortness of breath on exertion.

Moderate AMS produces severe headaches, not relieved by aspirin or ibuprofen, and persistent vomiting. The patient will complain of moderate fatigue.

Severe AMS (HAPE and HACE) is a life-threatening emergency. The patient will show changes in Consciousness and mental status. He may become ataxic (unable to walk straight), and severely fatigued and short of breath even at rest. The examiner may note a cough, possibly with gurgling respirations due to the accumulation of fluid in the lungs. The patient may appear cyanotic (blue or pale) and much weaker then others in the group.

The symptoms of Severe AMS can be confused or mixed with those of other problems such as hypoglycemia (low blood sugar), dehydration, hypothermia, hyperthermia, and exercise exhaustion. All of these problems can cause a decrease in muscular performance and efficiency. All can cause changes in Level of Consciousness and mental status. Under most field conditions, the most practical approach is to include all five problems as possible causes until proven otherwise.

➡️ *Treatment of AMS:* This is where two days of prevention is worth 4000 feet of cure. The key is to recognize the mild form of Altitude Sickness and allow your body time to adapt.

Mild AMS is treated with mild pain relievers such as aspirin, ibuprofen, or tylenol. The patient should avoid sedatives like alcohol or narcotic drugs which can depress respiration. This is the time to rest at the present altitude, or descend to a lower altitude until the body adapts. Diamox, available by prescription, is occasionally used to increase the rate of respiration by changing blood pH (consult a physician about its use).

Moderate AMS is treated with pain medication, rest, and avoidance of sedatives. In addition, an immediate descent of 1000–2000 feet is recommended, if possible. The patient should be observed closely for increasing severity of symptoms. Be prepared for an emergency descent if symptoms worsen. Supplemental oxygen and steroids (by physician's prescription) may be helpful if available.

Severe AMS is treated using all the techniques covered under the mild and moderate forms, *plus* an immediate descent of 2000–4000 feet. The Generic Treatment for Respiratory Distress (Chapter 4) should be followed. Exertion should be minimized, but there should be no delay in descent.

Field Treatment Summary
For Altitude Sickness

Mild AMS—Rest until Adapted, Pain Medication.

Moderate AMS—Descend 1000–2000 feet.

Severe AMS—Descend 2000–4000 feet.

COMMON
MEDICAL
PROBLEMS

15

ABDOMINAL PAIN

The word abdomen is a derivation of the Latin for "hidden," and rightly so. Everything that goes on inside the abdomen is well hidden from our eyes and can become the subject of a lot of conjecture and consternation. How do you know if your crew member's belly pain is from a developing appendicitis, or an undeveloped ability to digest whole grain? Should you call a passing ship for a lift back to Portland, or stick it out until you reach Bermuda?

Few symptoms can cause as much unnecessary grief as abdominal pain. Even experienced surgeons using a variety of diagnostic tests and tools have a difficult time figuring out what's going on inside a sore abdomen. Don't feel too bad if you can't figure it out either. Focus instead on the question: Is this pain likely to be caused by a serious problem?

For our purposes, we can consider the abdomen to be hiding three major components: hollow organs like the stomach and intestines, solid organs such as the liver and spleen, and the abdominal lining called the "peritoneum." Hollow organs contain digestive fluids and have muscular walls which contract rhythmically to move these fluids along the digestive system. Solid organs have a variety of functions and associated diseases, but in the field, we worry mostly about their potential for traumatic rupture and severe bleeding.

The peritoneum is a membrane that lines all of the organs and the abdominal wall inside the body cavity, normally isolated from digestive enzymes and bacteria. It is exquisitely sensitive to irritation from things like blood, bacteria, and digestive fluids which have entered the cavity through injury or illness. The peritoneum also represents a large surface area which, when irritated, can leak a large volume of fluid in a short period of time. Shock can rapidly develop.

Assessment of Abdominal Pain: Most abdominal pain is caused by the stretching of the hollow organs of the digestive system. This occurs when they are distended by gas or food while attempting their normal, rhythmic muscular contractions. This produces the crampy pain which precedes a bout of diarrhea or flatulence, after which you feel a whole lot better. The problem is well contained within the intestine and, when relieved, the system returns to normal.

Another source of benign abdominal discomfort is abdominal wall pain. This is associated with the musculature of the abdomen rather than any internal organs. It can usually be attributed to exertion. This type of pain will be relieved by rest, and made worse by movement.

Real problems begin when whatever is happening in the abdomen begins to affect the Circulatory System. This usually comes in the form of severe fluid loss from continued vomiting or diarrhea. Even more devastating is perforation of a hollow organ which releases it's contents into the abdominal cavity. This will inflame the peritoneum with subsequent severe pain, volume shock, and death.

Blunt trauma to the abdomen can cause severe bleeding from a ruptured solid organ, leading to shock. This should be anticipated in cases of persistent abdominal pain following injury. It can develop almost immediately, or become evident only after the peritoneum becomes irritated by free blood in the abdominal cavity.

Symptoms of peritoneal irritation from whatever cause are to be considered serious. These symptoms are included in the "RED FLAGS" of abdominal pain.

RED FLAGS = Potentially Serious Problems

—fever
—blood by mouth or rectum
—persistent vomiting or diarrhea
—pain persisting more than twelve hours
—tenderness (to the touch)
—signs of volume shock
—pain becoming worse following trauma

The presence of RED FLAG signs in abdominal pain does not always guarantee serious problems. It just means that the chances are high enough to warrant an evacuation.

Treatment of Abdominal Pain: Treat the cause. This usually means that you can't fix it in the field. Whether you're a surgeon or a woodcutter, *RED FLAGS = Evacuation.* You should continue to monitor the patient during transport and note any changes in condition. In the long-term care setting, abdominal pain or the accompanying RED FLAGS may resolve revealing the problem to be less serious. Its always better to cancel or slow down an evacuation in progress, rather than to start one too late.

16

CHEST PAIN

Just about anybody who enters a hospital emergency department, and uses the words "chest" and "pain" in the same sentence gets treated as if they are having a heart attack. It happens even though medical practitioners know that there are many causes of chest pain that have nothing to do with the heart. They recognize that the risk and expense involved in testing for heart attack is much lower than the risk and expense involved in failing to detect one. For the hospital, the choice is easy and the policy is clear. Unfortunately, this does not translate very well for the remote environment. We need a much better indication of the real potential for a heart problem to balance against the hazards of evacuation.

Assessment of Chest Pain: Just like the hospital, we look for a reasonable explanation for the pain. This may include heart problems. More often, however, it will be attributable to one of a number of other possibilities.

The most common cause of chest pain in the backcountry setting is muscle or rib pain from exercise or injury. This type of pain can usually be reproduced by movement. There is often a tender area in the same spot where the patient complains of pain. It is usually relieved by rest and aspirin or ibuprofen. The patient does not usually appear otherwise sick, or short of breath.

Chest pain from respiratory infection or lung injury will usually have a pretty clear history of preceding illness or injury. It may be accompanied by cough, fever, and sore throat. It is usually made worse by coughing and deep breathing. The patient is usually somewhat ill in appearance. This pain may be part of a serious Respiratory System problem, but not an indication of heart attack.

The pain associated with indigestion is usually accompanied by burping, heart burn, and nausea. Unlike the pain of heart attack, it is relieved by antacids. The patient will often give a long-standing history of similar episodes associated with certain foods or stress.

The chest pain of a heart attack is caused by ischemia (inadequate perfusion) of the heart muscle. It is typically described as being in the middle of the chest radiating to the jaw and left arm. The pain is often referred to as "crushing or constricting." There may be shortness of breath and sweating. Vital signs may show an irregular heart beat and the signs of shock (see page 67).

At least this is what the textbook says. Unfortunately, the classic pattern does not occur in all cases of heart attack. It can be mistaken for indigestion, respiratory infection, or chest-wall pain. In fact, the patient will be trying very hard to mistake it for anything but heart attack. If there is no other obvious cause, we must assume that chest pain represents a serious medical problem, especially when associated with RED FLAGS:

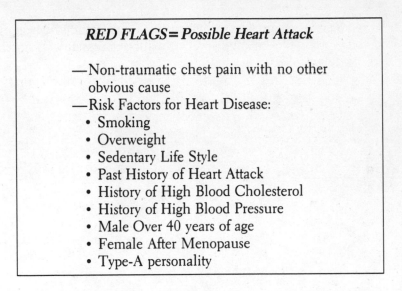

RED FLAGS = Possible Heart Attack

—Non-traumatic chest pain with no other
  obvious cause
—Risk Factors for Heart Disease:
  • Smoking
  • Overweight
  • Sedentary Life Style
  • Past History of Heart Attack
  • History of High Blood Cholesterol
  • History of High Blood Pressure
  • Male Over 40 years of age
  • Female After Menopause
  • Type-A personality

This does not mean that your slim, mellow, non-smoking, athletic, 20-year-old girlfriend can't have heart problems. It just means that it is very unlikely, and you are unlikely to call for a heroic evacuation with that thought in mind.

But, if your chest-pain patient is your overweight, two-pack-a-day-smoking, 45-year-old law firm partner, you'd best get him out of the woods. This does not mean he *is* having a heart attack, but the likelihood is high enough to justify evacuation.

Treatment of Suspected Heart Attack

1. Basic Life Support
2. Rest and Reassurance
3. Oxygen if Available
4. Evacuation—quick, but not stressful.
5. Medication—If the patient has medication, assist him in taking it according to his directions.

17

DIARRHEA

One of the functions of the large intestine is to absorb fluid from feces just before excretion. This serves to conserve the body's fluid balance, and allow you some degree of control over when and where excretion occurs. Diarrhea develops when the lining of the intestinal space is irritated by infection or toxins and fails to absorb fluid. The intestine can, in addition, leak more body fluid on its own, contributing to general fluid loss.

Assessment of Diarrhea: Like abdominal pain, what we want to know is this: serious or not serious? Diarrhea which is a softer version of normal stool, and relatively infrequent in an otherwise healthy individual, is usually nothing to worry about. Even if it lasts for several days or weeks, fluid losses can be replaced by oral intake.

Diarrhea can be a symptom of other, more serious problems (see Chapter 15). Diarrhea itself becomes a real problem when fluid loss occurs so rapidly that it cannot be replaced by drinking and eating.

RED FLAGS = Potentially Serious Problems

—persistent, more than twenty-four hours
—signs of volume shock
—blood in stool
—fever
—persistent pain (see Abdominal Pain)

Treatment of Diarrhea: Diarrhea which does not show Red-Flag signs can sometimes be helped by bismuth subsalicylate (Pepto-Bismol) or similar over-the-counter preparations. But, most importantly, you should pay attention to replacing fluid losses with oral intake. Using juice, or water with a touch of salt and sugar, will replace some body electrolytes. Time will usually correct the situation, but if the problem persists longer than a week, medical advice should be sought.

When the RED FLAG signs are noted, evacuation should be initiated. If signs of volume shock are present, it is an emergency. Replacement fluids should be given by mouth as much as the patient can tolerate. Use dilute juice, or a solution of water with a pinch of salt and sugar per quart.

18

CONSTIPATION

Constipation is usually the result of the large intestine doing just what it's supposed to do: absorb fluid from feces. If you are dehydrated, fluid recovery can turn feces into something resembling metamorphic rock. This can be tough for even the most energetic hollow-organ muscle contractions to deal with.

Assessment of Constipation: We are told by the advertising media that at least one well formed stool a day is the birthright of every human being. Less than that, and our diet and lifestyle is all wrong. They may have a point, but such time limits are a little unrealistic in the backcountry.

Constipation starts to become annoying when you feel bad because of it. Constipation represents a real problem when the rest of the body begins to suffer (see Chapter 15). Exactly when this occurs is highly individual. Some people can go nine days before being bothered by the lack of a bowel movement, while others become cranky after only twenty-four hours.

Prevention of Constipation: Maintaining fluid balance by staying well hydrated will make it unnecessary for the large intestine to absorb too much fluid from feces. A good indicator for hydration is urine production. You should be drinking enough fluid to be producing light yellow colored urine fairly frequently.

Take the time and find the privacy for a decent bowel movement. This is especially difficult on boats at sea in rough conditions, or on a big wall climb when relieving oneself becomes a life-threatening adventure. But, it is extremely important. If feces sit in the intestine long enough, metamorphosis will occur no matter how well hydrated you are.

Diets high in fiber create bulk which stimulates bowel contraction and retains water in the fecal material.

➡ *Treatment of Constipation*

Bulk agents like Metamucil and similar substances work like a high-fiber diet.

Osmotic Agents like Milk of Magnesia draw water into the intestine.

Lubricants like mineral oil taken by mouth will smooth intestinal and stool surfaces moving things along with less effort and pain.

Laxatives including Exlax, and bisocodyl (Dulcolax) suppositories can be used if the above fail. Bisocodyl is generally easier to use because it is a rectal stimulant and causes less cramping.

Enemas are generally viewed as a last resort. Giving warm water per rectum will hydrate and soften stool. The additional bulk will stimulate bowel contraction. Do not use an enema in the presence of RED FLAGS for abdominal pain.

19

NAUSEA AND VOMITING

Like diarrhea, vomiting can be the result of a problem with the gastrointestinal system, or be a symptom of other problems such as motion sickness, toxin ingestion, head injury, or infection. Finding and treating the primary cause is the priority. However, you must consider the additional problems that can be caused by severe fluid loss as well.

Assessment of Vomiting: Vomiting which is associated with RED FLAGS is considered serious. This includes sea sickness which is persistent and not responsive to medication, or persistent vomiting for any reason.

RED FLAGS for Vomiting

—fluid losses cannot be replaced by drinking
—associated with RED FLAGS for Abdominal Pain
—persistent, more than twenty-four hours

➡ Treatment of Vomiting

Replace Fluid Losses—As for diarrhea.

Protect Airway—Vomiting can cause airway obstruction or pulmonary edema if inhaled. Position the patient to allow drainage.

Evacuate—If vomiting is potentially serious.

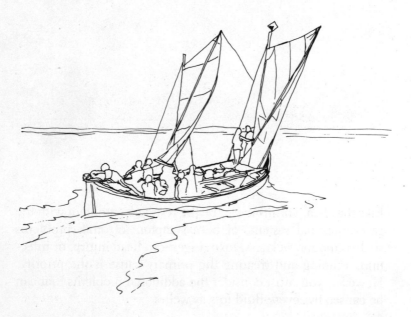

20

EAR PROBLEMS

EXTERNAL EAR INFECTION (Swimmer's Ear)

Swimmer's ear is an inflammation of the external audi-
tory canal. That is, the tube leading from the outside environment to the outside surface of the ear drum. The problem is
usually caused by bacteria which infect skin softened by prolonged soaking in water.

Assessment of Swimmer's Ear: Like any infection, it will be
characterized by redness, warmth, swelling, and pain. The external structures of the ear and surrounding area will be tender
to the touch, and the ear canal itself will be exquisitely sensitive. There is usually a history of recent and repetitive immersion in water.

➡ *Treatment of Swimmer's Ear:* The treatment of choice is antibiotic ear drops, available by physician's prescription. In lieu of that, regular cleansing of the ear canal with a Q-tip dipped in rubbing alcohol followed by mineral oil should reduce the amount of debris and bacteria and contribute to healing. Do not use dry Q-tips because they will further irritate the ear canal. Staying out of the water and allowing the ear to heal will help considerably.

MIDDLE EAR INFECTION AND SINUSITIS

The area referred to as the "middle ear" begins inside the ear drum and extends through a narrow opening into the nasal cavity. It is similar in structure to the other sinuses which are open spaces, lined by mucous membranes, with narrow openings into the nose. If anything obstructs the opening, the sinuses will fill with fluid. Sooner or later, bacteria will begin to grow in this fluid, producing an infection.

Assessment of Sinusitis: The typical sign of sinus infection is facial or ear pain. There will often be a history of several days of mild cold or flu symptoms with a stuffy or runny nose. Bending over at the waist increases pressure in the affected sinus or ear and generally increases the pain. Sinusitis, in the form of middle ear infection, can be differentiated from swimmer's ear by the fact that, although the ear hurts, the external ear structures and ear canal are not tender to touch. In more severe infections, you may see some discharge of green or yellow pus from the nose. Fever is another symptom of more serious infection, as is swelling or tenderness of the face.

➡ *Treatment of Sinusitis:* Like any abscess in a closed space, it can be improved by drainage. We can try to reduce the swelling and fluid obstructing the narrow openings to the nose to allow this to happen. Decongestant nasal spray, or breathing steam by holding your towel-draped head over a pot of hot water, is useful for this. Systemic decongestants such as Sudafed tablets may also help. Keeping yourself well hydrated is also important. This will allow mucous to remain fluid and mobile. Antibiotics are routinely used and are generally necessary for definitive treatment.

Middle-ear infections may drain themselves spontaneously by rupturing the ear drum. If this occurs, blood and pus may drain from the ear. If pain is relieved, and no fever develops, there is no emergency in this. Keep the ear dry and see your doctor when you get ashore.

21

NOSEBLEED

It doesn't take much trauma to rupture the blood vessels in the nose. The most easily injured ones are near the front of the nose (anterior). Blood from here will drain out of the nose if the patient is positioned upright with the head forward.

Assessment of Nosebleed: The problem here is to distinguish a simple nosebleed from something more significant. If the bleeding started spontaneously, or while blowing or picking your nose, you can be pretty sure it's not complicated. However, if the bleeding is the result of trauma, you must consider the possibility of facial bone fracture and head injury.

Treatment of Nosebleed: First, sit your patient down, and calm him down. Position him to allow for drainage out of the nose, then have him blow out any clots. This sounds scary, but it won't cause the bleeding to get worse. Now, you or the patient should pinch the nostrils together and hold firmly for fifteen minutes while sitting erect. This applies simple direct pressure to the most likely bleeding source. Remember, to stop the bleeding, it is essential to hold enough pressure for a long enough time. This should stop most of nosebleeds that you are likely to see. Bleeding from the nose might return over the next few hours, but the treatment simply needs to be repeated.

If you encounter the rare, persistent nosebleed in the field, your best response is the same as for any other bleeding which you are unable to control. Make the patient as comfortable and quiet as possible and send for help. Control the airway by positioning him face down, or on the side, with the chest and head supported to allow for drainage from the nose and mouth. Prepare for a carry-out evacuation.

22

URINARY-TRACT INFECTION

The female urethra is only a few centimeters long. It is fairly easy for normal skin surface bacteria to migrate from the outside into the normally sterile bladder. Once there, bacteria are able to reproduce rapidly and begin to invade and inflame the soft-tissue lining. Normally, frequent urination flushes bacteria out of the bladder and urethra, preventing this from happening.

In both the civilized and backcountry settings there are a number of ways that this system can be upset. Perhaps the most common to the wilderness traveler is urinary retention. This is usually due to slight dehydration. The body's normal efforts to preserve fluid results in low urine output, and infrequent flushing of the urinary tract. The same situation can occur simply through lack of opportunity to urinate, such as "holding it" until morning rather than getting out of a warm sleeping bag in the middle of the night. Either way, any bacteria entering the bladder and urethra have a longer period of time in which to multiply and invade the tissue lining.

Another common cause of urinary-tract infection in the female is inadequate hygiene. In settings where bathing is difficult or impossible the bacteria count on the outer surface of the skin increases dramatically. Add this to the habit of "drip drying" instead of using toilet paper and you have a greater opportunity for infection.

A third mechanism for infection is direct trauma to the urethra. The usual culprit is frequent or vigorous sexual activity, but it can also be caused by the seat of a mountain bike or a climbing harness. This is the so-called "honeymoon cystitis." The urethral opening becomes inflamed, is invaded by bacteria, and infection results.

More complicated and dangerous infections can develop when the bacteria climb beyond the bladder to invade the ureters and kidney. Sexually-transmitted diseases are also considered more dangerous because the bacteria or virus is foreign to the body and is more difficult to eradicate. *In the male, infection of the urinary tract is unusual, and always indicates a complicated condition. The most common cause is sexually-transmitted disease.*

Assessment of Urinary-Tract Infection: The classic symptoms of uncomplicated urinary-tract infection include low pelvic pain, frequent urination in small amounts, cloudy or blood-tinged urine, and pain, tingling, or burning on urination.

In the female, it is possible to confuse infection of the urinary tract with vaginal infection. Inflammation of the vagina and external genitalia can also cause pain and burning on urination (see Vaginitis). Pain and burning on urination in the male is usually due to sexually-transmitted disease.

Symptoms which indicate that infection has progressed beyond the superficial lining of the urethra and bladder can include any of the symptoms above plus RED FLAGS:

RED FLAGS IN UTI = Serious Problem

—fever
—back pain and tenderness (kidney involvement)
—Urinary-tract infection in the male
—Sexually-transmitted disease

Treatment of Urinary-Tract Infection: The treatment for
early urinary-tract infection includes the use of antibiotics.
The patient should seek medical care for this purpose. Temporary measures, pending evacuation, involve treating UTI like
any other soft-tissue infection with drainage and cleansing.
Keep the external genitalia as clean as possible. Drink plenty
of fluids to irrigate the infection. You can also try vitamin C
orally, 1 gram 4 times a day. Vitamin C is an acid (ascorbic
acid) and only a small amount can be absorbed by the body at
a time. The excess is excreted in the urine, making it too
acidic to harbor most strains of bacteria. Symptoms of UTI accompanied by RED FLAGS indicate a possibly serious problem. Infection of the kidneys can become a life-threatening
condition.

23

VAGINITIS

Inflammation and infection of the vagina often occurs when something upsets the normal ecological balance between yeast and bacteria allowing one of the species to grow out of control. For example, taking penicillin for a strep throat will kill many of the bacteria in the vagina as well. This opens the way for an overgrowth of yeast, which is not affected by penicillin. Changes in the vaginal environment caused by clothing, sexual activity, stress, and other factors can upset this balance as well. Because of frequently hot, humid conditions, vaginitis is common in the backcountry.

Assessment of Vaginitis: Vaginitis typically causes itching or burning, and a whitish or "cheesy" vaginal discharge. There may also be tingling or burning as urine irritates inflamed tissues, causing some confusion with urinary-tract infection.

Treatment of Vaginitis: Temporary reduction of symptoms pending medical attention may be obtained by using a douche of betadine solution diluted to 0.025% (one teaspoon of betadine in a quart of water) used daily. An alternative douche solution may be prepared by diluting 1 tablespoon of vinegar in 1 quart of water. A douche should not be used by a pregnant patient. The situation can also be improved by a dry and cool environment. This means wearing loose-fitting clothing and spending less time in the wet suit.

── 24 ──

RESPIRATORY INFECTION

The "common cold," with its stuffy nose, sore throat, runny eyes, and cough has been harassing people since people began. There is no reason to believe that it won't pick on you, expedition or no expedition. You should be ready to deal with it.

The mild respiratory infections that we label "colds" or "flu" are caused by viruses. They produce a multiplicity of symptoms which conspire to keep us miserable until our body's immune system identifies the bug, produces specific antibodies, and eradicates it. Problems develop when the virus is particularly virulent, or the viral infection opens the way for a secondary bacterial infection to take hold. This is how people who start with a cold can end up with pneumonia, bronchitis, or strep throat.

Assessment of Upper Respiratory Infection: Mild upper respiratory infection is characterized by runny nose, mild headache, sneezing, coughing, tearing eyes, mild sore throat, muscular aches, and low-grade fever (below 102°F). Other than being slightly annoyed and uncomfortable, the patient is usually not significantly impaired in her ability to perform normal tasks.

Significant respiratory disease may have been preceded by the above symptoms, or develop independently. In serious respiratory infections coughing typically becomes productive of thick yellow, green, or brown sputum ("coughing in colors"). The patient may experience fevers and chills, shortness of breath, and chest pain on respiration.

➡️ *Treatment of Upper Respiratory Infection:* The treatment of mild upper respiratory infection involves making the patient more comfortable while the body works to defeat the virus. Use whatever over-the-counter medications make the patient feel better, while not interfering with their ability to function. Local decongestants such as nasal sprays, systemic decongestants, and non-narcotic cough medications are very helpful. So is aspirin.

Equally important is maintaining fluid balance, eating well, staying warm, and getting enough rest. This reduces the number of stressors that the body has to deal with. The system will then be free to focus on fighting the virus, and preventing a secondary bacterial invasion. The patient who is "coughing in colors" generally requires antibiotics and further medical care.

25

DENTAL PROBLEMS

Teeth become a problem when they are fractured or avulsed (knocked out) by trauma. They become a nightmare when infected. Not only is there pain, but the pain can interfere with eating and drinking, which is essential to survival. Anyone contemplating an extended wilderness trip, or ocean passage, should have any potential dental problems attended to before departure.

Assessment of Dental Trauma: First recognize that loose teeth, or pieces of teeth, can result in airway obstruction. Damage to teeth can be associated with head and neck injury. Pain can produce Acute Stress Reaction. Swallowing blood can cause vomiting.

Assessment of dental trauma is directed at ensuring that potential BIG 3 problems are considered and stabilized. Beyond that, broken teeth do not represent a medical emergency.

➡️ ***Treatment of Dental Trauma:*** First, remove avulsed or fractured teeth that might obstruct the airway. While protecting the cervical spine, position the patient to allow drainage of blood and debris from the mouth, rather than down the throat. Examine the patient to rule out other BIG 3 problems such as head or neck injury.

If the patient is stable and alert, have him rinse his mouth with cool water. This will clean out blood clots and loose teeth and help to stop bleeding. Examine the mouth with a flashlight. Look for teeth that are loose or fractured but still in the socket. Look for empty sockets that could match any avulsed teeth you may have found.

Teeth which have been cleanly avulsed (knocked out) have a fair chance of reattaching if returned to their socket within an hour or so—the sooner the better. Try not to handle the tooth by its roots, which will disturb the attachment fibers. Rinse the tooth in clean water and push it gently all the way back into its socket. You can sometimes splint the tooth to a solid one adjacent to it by tying it with dental floss or fishing line. Any teeth which are very loose, but still in the socket, may be splinted in this manner as well.

Fractured teeth which are still in place are often extremely sensitive on exposure to air if the nerve is still alive. The open site can be treated with topical oral pain relievers and covered temporarily with dental wax or Cavit. Cavit is a temporary filling material which hardens on exposure to saliva. Ask your dentist about acquiring some for your first-aid kit.

The loss of a filling can be treated the same way using wax or Cavit to protect the sensitive nerve tissue that is exposed when the filling falls out. The patient should eat only soft foods and cool liquids until seen by a dentist.

Assessment of Dental Infection: "Toothache" usually describes the pain experienced when an infection develops inside the tooth and at the base of the root. Bacteria enters through a break in the enamel caused by trauma or a cavity, and form an abscess with the typical local inflammation, warmth, and pain. Swelling of the gum on the affected side may be evident as well as tenderness of one or more teeth when tapped with a finger or stick.

The infection may remain localized, or spread into the adjacent bone or sinus. In either case, it will be extremely uncomfortable. Both the infection and the pain it causes will be difficult to manage in the field.

Treatment of Dental Infection: The treatment of a dental infection includes drainage, antibiotics, and pain relief. Up until quite recently in dental history, drainage was invariably performed by pulling the tooth. The preferred method today is drilling and cleaning the inside of the tooth, and installing a filling. Antibiotics are often used to bring the infection under control and pain relievers are usually necessary. What this means to you in the field is as simple as it is unfortunate: you need a dentist. Temporary pain relief may be obtained with oral topical pain relievers and aspirin or ibuprofen.

26

EYE PROBLEMS

The common term "red eye" refers to inflammation of the thin, membranous lining of the eye and the inside of the eye lids (conjunctiva). The cause of the inflammation may be infection, sunburn, sand in the eye, trauma, chemical irritation, or even fatigue. It can also represent one of the symptoms of a more serious condition like glaucoma.

Assessment of Red Eye: All the various types of red eye produce similar symptoms. The patient will complain of an itching or burning sensation, tearing, and photophobia (discomfort caused by bright lights). The white of the eye will be covered with the enlarged blood vessels of the inflamed conjunctiva. In milder cases, the cornea will remain clear. The pupil will continue to react to light. Vision will be unaffected except for transient blurring caused by tears or yellow exudate. Normal eye movements will be uncomfortable, but fully intact.

In more severe cases there may be clouding of the cornea, persistent visual disturbances, and severe headache. Causes of red eye include:

Foreign Body—Sand or other debris which gets onto the conjunctiva will cause immediate irritation, redness, and tearing. Onset is usually abrupt, and the cause often obvious.

Corneal Abrasion—The clear center structure of the eye can be scratched by a foreign body, branch, fingernail, or wind-blown ice crystals. It is exquisitely sensitive and will cause considerable pain and inflammation. Larger abrasions can be seen on the surface of the cornea on examination. Corneal abrasions can cause a "foreign body sensation" making the patient feel like there is something in the eye.

Sunburn—Ultraviolet light can burn the conjunctiva and cornea as it does the unprotected skin. The result is the same: pain, redness, and sometimes swelling. Exam will reveal that the inflammation is limited to the sun-exposed part of the eye, leaving the conjunctiva under the lids unaffected. In severe cases, the cornea may become pitted and cloudy in appearance.

Infection—This is what most practitioners mean by the term "conjunctivitis." Bacteria invade the conjunctiva causing the typical signs and symptoms of infection. The patient may notice yellow exudate which can stick the eyelids together during sleep. The eyelids themselves may appear slightly puffy and reddened.

Chemical Irritation—Soap, dirty contact lenses, stove fuel, and other irritants can cause chemical conjunctivitis. In mild cases, the cornea remains clear. In severe cases it may be pitted or cloudy in appearance.

➡ **Treatment of Red Eye:** Mild inflammation is usually easily treated in the field. If the cause is known, correct it, and/or protect it, and allow it to heal.

Foreign Body—The easiest and least traumatic way to remove something from the eye is by irrigation with water. The simplest way to accomplish this is to have the patient immerse his face in clean water and blink his eyes. If there's no lake or stream handy, irrigate with your water bottle. Position him on his side with the affected eye up. Pour water gently on the lateral end of the eye and let it run across the eye toward the nose. Holding the lids open is not necessary if the patient can continue to blink during irrigation.

This technique will remove almost any object that lands in the eye. If the patient continues to have the sensation of something in there, you'll have to go looking for it. Gently pull the lids away from the eye one at a time while the patient looks in all directions. Look on the eye itself as well as on the conjunctival surface of the inside of the eye lids. A flashlight helps.

If you find something, use a wet cotton swab or corner of a gauze pad to lift it off the membrane. If the object is imbedded in the conjunctiva or cornea and resists your efforts to remove it, leave it alone. Imbedded foreign bodies require medical attention. Patch the eye, if safe to do so, and plan to walk out. Beware, however, of using a patch in situations where impaired vision could be dangerous. Depth perception is lost when one eye is patched. Be careful walking anyone whose vision is impaired.

Corneal Abrasion—If the foreign body sensation persists but you are unable to find anything, the problem may be a corneal abrasion or scratch on the conjunctiva left by the dislodged foreign body. Sometimes the abrasion will be visible on careful examination. This will usually resolve on its own over the course of twenty-four hours. A patch should be used if it makes the patient more comfortable, and the reduction of vision can be tolerated safely.

Sunburn—Most inflammation from ultraviolet (UV) exposure is mild and self limiting. However, if the damage is severe enough to cause cloudiness of the cornea or snowblindness, the eyes must be placed at rest and allowed to heal. Fortunately UV rays do not penetrate deeply, so damage is usually superficial.

The treatment involves patching both eyes (like the treatment for corneal abrasion), and keeping the patient rested and quiet. Pain medication may be necessary. Symptoms should resolve within 24–48 hours. This is the time to be bivouaced, not stumbling blindly down a glacier to find a helicopter.

Infection—Most bacterial and viral conjunctivitis is self-limiting, but this is difficult to predict. Like any infected tissue, allow the eyes to drain. Do not use a patch because this will prevent drainage of bacteria. Some relief may be obtained using frequent rinsing and warm soaks. Treatment with antibiotics is usually necessary, especially if symptoms appear to become progressively worse, rather than stabilizing or improving. Note also that a conjunctival infection can be quite contagious. Avoid sharing towels, goggles, or face masks.

Chemical Irritation—The treatment for chemical exposure is irrigation, and lots of it (30 minutes minimum). Expect mild redness following prolonged irrigation, but it should begin to resolve within several hours following treatment. If it gets worse, the chemical may still be present. Irrigation should be repeated and evacuation plans made.

SECTION VII

WILDERNESS RESCUE

About a week ago, I took a break from writing to climb Bigelow Mountain with my old friend, and a new physician, Don Jackel. The autumn leaves were unusually beautiful in the subdued light of a cold rain. The trail was wet and slick forcing us to keep our eyes to the ground as much as on the scenery. But this was familiar country to both of us and we made good time.

As we climbed, I couldn't help but think over recently drafted parts of this book. At one point, I stopped on a steeply sloping section of the trail and asked Don, "What would you do if I broke a leg right here?" Being fresh out of medical school and an experienced outdoorsman, the answers came easily. That is, up to the part about leaving me here to go get help.

Shelter would be necessary. The temperature was in the low 40s with a steady rain, forecast to become snow. The forest was thick and saturated, and the slope too steep to pitch a tent. The nearest flat spot was about 100 feet uphill. It was already late afternoon.

This was only northern New England, not Antarctica or Greenland. We were within four miles of the trailhead, but could have had serious problems all the same. I was reminded of a phrase I frequently use with my Outward Bound students: "Nobody said this was going to be easy."

Don eventually came up with the idea of building a low platform of branches between two nearby trees with the tent fly pitched overhead. I would then, somehow, be placed on the platform, on my foam pad, in my sleeping bag, with the stove, water, and food near at hand.

The plan sounded feasible, and we had all the necessary twine and tools to do it. We estimated that it would take about an hour and a half to accomplish. His hike out would take another two hours, and a carry-out evacuation about five hours to organize. I could expect to seem him again just about sunrise.

I returned to my writing to realize how many times treatment plans call for "evacuation to medical care," as if it were as easy as catching a bus. In reality, it is everything but easy, especially when the injured person is no longer able to walk. The problem is compounded by the unavailability of trained and experienced wilderness rescue teams in much of the world.

Outside of state and national parks there is little in the way of organized municipal response to backcountry emergencies. The responsibility for wilderness rescue is assumed by a variety of officials depending on where you are. This might include the Warden Service, Coast Guard, local fire departments, police, or ambulance crews. The official response usually relies heavily on volunteer rescue teams, the National Guard, ski patrols, and other organizations and individuals to do the actual work.

In some cases, your rescue will be a well coordinated effort by competent officials and well trained volunteers. In others, the effort can be disorganized, inefficient, and downright dangerous. Either can happen depending on where you are, the situation you're in, and even the day of the week.

In spite of this inconsistency, it is not a situation which merits much complaint. As backcountry travelers, we represent a minuscule portion of the general population. It is difficult to justify maintaining a sophisticated and expensive wilderness rescue system for so few people.

To enter the wilderness is to accept a much greater degree of personal responsibility. We must be able to get outselves out of trouble whenever possible. Lacking that, we must be able to be of the greatest possible assistance to those who are coming to help us.

PREPARATION

The traditional view holds "The best preparation for medical emergencies is not to have them in the first place." There are plenty of how-to books on camping, sailing, canoeing, ice climbing, and so forth to help you do it right. Read them.

Since having medical emergencies is what *this* book is about, I'll take the statement a step further: "The best time to have a medical emergency is when you're ready for it." Being ready means having the right attitude, knowledge, equipment, and margin of safety for the expedition you're planning.

Attitude, in my view, is the way one relates with the forces of the natural world. It is so much more peaceful to flow with natural trends, than push against them. However, it is not always possible to go down river, down hill, downwind, or with the tide. We tend to have schedules, destinations, and personal goals that put us in confrontation with nature.

Of course, challenging the elements can be great fun and an exhilarating experience. As long as you continue to feel that way, you'll be OK. However, one must beware of developing an adverse relationship with nature. This is a forewarning of serious trouble.

When it starts raining on *you*, or the wind shifts just to make *you* angry, or the snow starts just because *it* knows you're almost at the summit, your attitude has become dangerous. In an emergency situation, a bad attitude is big trouble. It contributes to irrational behavior, poor judgment, and despair. When you feel the "attitude," its time to change your plans and re-establish harmony with your surroundings.

Knowing how to handle medical emergencies is a product of both information and experience. Only by combining the two, can you gain real competence in the art of wilderness medicine. The information is readily available in this book, and others like it. The experience is more difficult to come by. A reasonable substitute, at least as a beginning, can be found in the form of a quality hands-on course taught for the backcountry setting.

Knowing what to expect of the environment you are entering is important too. What is the weather and terrain like? How far will you be from help, if needed? What kind of help is available? Whom do you contact? Where are shelters, ranger stations, roads, water, and so forth located?

Equipment for wilderness emergency care is surprisingly simple. The real first-aid kit is your knowledge and experience. The bandages, ointments, moleskin, and other items in your pack (see Appendix) are just tools for minor maintenance and repair.

How much first-aid equipment you carry is a function of how you carry it, how many people you're responsible for, where you're going, and what you know. There is no point in carrying anything you don't know how to use. If you're carrying it on your back, there is no reason to carry anything which can be improvised from something else. As a result, the average backpacker's first-aid kit is very small and simple. Larger groups, or people traveling by vehicle, boat, or horse have the luxury of carrying more complete supplies.

The margin of safety in wilderness travel is the most important factor of all. When I stopped to question Don about my theoretical broken leg, we were well within our margin of safety for that situation. We were dry, warm, and well fed. Our tent and sleeping bags were dry, and we had enough food, water, and fuel. We were prepared to spend another night out if necessary.

Had we allowed ourselves to get wet, chilled, and low on supplies, the situation would be entirely different. Breaking a leg at that point could easily be fatal. This is so often the case near the end of an expedition when fatigue has set in, supplies are low, and common sense flies to the moon.

When you're in the mountains, out to sea, or on the river, you should frequently ask yourself "what would I do if something went wrong?" This is a great exercise for the traveler new to the backcountry. If your answers are not coming up clear and reasonable, you are beyond your margin of safety.

As you gain experience, your awareness of your own margin of safety becomes part of you. You feel comfortable within it, and uneasy outside it. Pushing your own limits then becomes a matter of choice, rather than accident.

COMMUNICATION

When you have stabilized a medical problem as best you can, and have decided that outside help will be required, your communication skill becomes critical. Presenting a clear picture of the situation will allow rescuers to best apply their own local knowledge, experience, and resources to helping you solve your problem. This is where your SOAP note really becomes valuable. Not only has it helped you organize your thoughts, it can now provide the basis for organizing an evacuation. This is true whether you communicate by radio, telephone, carrier pigeon, or by sending a runner with a note.

Along with your SOAP note, you should include information about the scene. Describe the general condition of the group, weather and terrain conditions, and the status of food supplies and shelter. Try to stick to facts as much as possible. Avoid value judgments like: "oh my God, it's really bad, come quick!" These provide no useful information, and only distract people from a good planning process.

Recognize that any good rescue team is trained to perform their own assessment of the scene and the patient's condition. Their assessment may differ from yours. Work with them, pointing out elements of your assessment that will help form a reasonable plan. This is no time for arguing. In all but the most unusual cases, when you've asked for rescue the rescuers are in charge.

EVACUATION

Responding to a medical emergency can be done by bringing the medical resources to the patient, or the patient to the medicine. Usually, it is a combination of the two. For example, rescue teams may bring intravenous fluids and oxygen to assist in stabilizing a patient during the carry-out. For the most part, though, the patient needs to return to civilization for definitive care.

The urgency with which this happens is a function of the patient's condition and the resources and skills available. It also hinges on your ability to distinguish real emergencies from logistical dilemmas. Very few backcountry situations really justify an all-out rapid evacuation. Only those injuries which involve a BIG 3 system in a big way, deserve a big evacuation. Anything else can be more controlled, less desperate, and a lot less trouble.

APPENDICES

PERSONAL FIRST AID KIT—SUGGESTED CONTENTS

Materials:
- 6—alcohol swabs
- 1—roll 1" tape
- 4—4" × 4" gauze pads
- 1—8" × 7½" bulk dressing
- 1—3" gauze roll
- 1—4" elastic bandage
- 10—band-aids
- 1—3" × 6" blister pad, e.g. Spenco Adhesive Knit, or moleskin
- 1 pr.—examination gloves
- 2—cotton-tipped applicators
- 6—blanket pins
- 1—low-reading clinical thermometer
- 1—#11 scalpel blade
- 1 pr.—fine tweezers
- 1—emergency flashlight
- 1—lighter or waterproof matches
- 1—knife
- 1—small container of liquid soap
- 1—container of 2% tincture of iodine
- 1—tube of antibiotic ointment
- 1—container of total sun block

Medication (Non-Prescription):
- small bottle of aspirin, ibuprofen, or Tylenol
- small bottle of dental analgesic, e.g. Orabase

stool softener, e.g. Colase
laxatives: pills or suppositories
package of Pepto-Bismol tablets
package of antacid tablets
cough and cold preparations as desired

WATER PURIFICATION

There are three acceptable methods:
1. **Boil**: 10 minutes. Add 1 minute for each 1000 feet above sea level.
2. **Chemicals**:
    a. *Iodine Tincture (2%)*—Use 5 drops of tincture per quart of water and let it stand for 30 minutes. Double the time if the water is cold. Double the dose if the water is cloudy.
    b. *Iodine Tablets*—One tablet per quart of water and let it stand for 30 minutes. Double the time if the water is cold. Double the dose if the water is cloudy.
3. **Filters**: To prevent clogging, pre-filter the water through a cloth to remove large sediment. Note: The typical .2 micron filter does not remove viruses (e.g., hepatitis).

GLOSSARY

Common Abbreviations

AMPLE Allergies
Medicines
Past history of medical
problems
Last meal
Events leading up
to injury

AVPU Alert
Verbal stimulus
response
Painful stimulus
response
Unresponsive

ALS   Advanced Life Support

BLS   Basic Life Support

C   Level of Consciousness

CNS   Central Nervous System

CPR   Cardio-pulmonary
      resuscitation

CSM   Circulation, Sensation,
      Movement

HACE High Altitude Cerebral
      Edema

HAPE High Altitude
      Pulmonary Edema

Hx   History

ICP   Intracranial Pressure

IV   Intravenous

MAST Military Anti-Shock
      Garment

MI   Myocardial Infarction
      (heart attack)

MOI   Mechanism Of Injury

MS   Mental Status

O_2 Oxygen

PAS   Patient Assessment
      System

PFA   Pain-Free Activity

RF   Red Flag

RICE Rest
      Ice

Compression
Elevation

Rx   Treatment

SOB   Shortness Of Breath

SOAP Subjective—Information
      gained by questioning
      Objective—Information
      gathered during examina-
      tion of the patient
      Assessment—List of
      problems discovered
      Plan—What is to be done

TIP   Traction Into Position

S/SX Signs/Symptoms

VS   Vital Signs (with time
      recorded)
      BP—Blood Pressure
      R—Respiratory Rate
      T— Core Temperature
      C—Level of Conscious
      ness, (Mental Status
      if Alert)
      S—Skin
      P—Pulse

Glossary

Abrasion: Superficial wound which damages only the outermost layers of skin or cornea.

Abscess: An infection which has been isolated from the rest of the body by inflammation.

Ace Bandage, ™: The brand name of an elastic bandage used to apply compression to an injured extremity.

Acute Stress Reaction (ASR): Autonomic Nervous system controlled response to stress which can cause severe, but temporary and reversible changes in vital signs. ASR can be sympathetic or parasympathetic.

Airway: The passage for air movement from the nose and mouth through the throat to the lungs.

Airway, lower: trachea, bronchi, alveoli

Airway, upper: Mouth, nose, throat (larynx)

Altitude sickness: Also known as Acute Mountain Sickness (AMS). The combined effects of oxygen deprivation at high elevations. Can be mild, moderate, or severe.

Alveoli: Membranous air sacks in the lungs where gas is exchanged with the blood.

Anaphylaxis: Systematic allergic reaction involving generalized edema of all body surfaces and vascular shock.

"Anticipated Problems" (A'): Problems which may develop over time as a result of injury, illness, or the environment.

Aspiration: Inhaling foreign liquid or other material into the lungs.

Basic Life Support (BLS): The generic process of supporting the functions of the Circulatory, Respiratory, and Nervous systems using artificial ventilations, chest compressions, bleeding control, and manual spinal immobilization.

Blood Pressure Cuff: Also known as a sphygmomanometer. Used for measuring blood pressure.

Cardiac arrest: Loss of effective heart activity.

Cardiogenic shock: Shock due to inadequate pumping action of the heart.

Cardio-Pulmonary Resuscitation (CPR): A technique for artificially circulating oxygenated blood in the absence of effective heart activity. Includes artificial respiration and chest compressions.

Capillaries: The smallest blood vessels in body tissues where gasses and nutrients are exchanged between tissue cells and the circulating blood.

Cartilage: Connective tissue on the ends of bones at joints which provide a smooth gliding surface.

Carotid pulse: The pulse felt on the side of the neck at the site of the carotid artery.

Cavit, ™: The brand name of a temporary dental filling material which hardens on exposure to saliva.

Central Nervous System: The brain and spinal cord.

CVA (Cerebrovascular Accident): Brain problem caused by ischemia due to the rupture or clotting of a blood vessel in the brain.

Cervical spine: The section of the spine in the neck between the base of the skull and the top of the thorax.

Cold Challenge: The combined cooling influence of wind, humidity, and ambient temperature.

Cold response: The normal body response, including the shell/core effect of shivering, to the cold challenge.

Compartment syndrome: Swelling within a confined body compartment which develops enough pressure to prevent adequate perfusion and results in death of tissue (necrosis).

Compensation: Involuntary changes in body function designed to maintain perfusion of vital body tissue in the presence of injury or illness.

Conjunctiva: The membrane covering the white of the eye and the inner surfaces of the eyelids.

Conjunctivitis: Inflammation of the conjunctiva due to irritation, infection, or injury. Also known as "Red Eye."

Level of Consciousness: Describes the level of brain function in terms of responsiveness to specific stimuli (the APVU Scale): A = Alert, V = responds to verbal stimuli, P = responds to painful stimuli, U = Unresponsive to any stimuli.

Cornea: The clear part of the eye over the iris and the pupil.

Cornice: An overhanging drift of snow formed as wind blows over a ridge or mountaintop.

Decompensation: Failure of compensation mechanisms.

Dental abscess: Infection at the base of a tooth.

Diagnosis: The specific identification of an illness or injury by name.

Diaphragm: Muscle at the lower end of the chest cavity

which, when contracting, creates a vacuum which draws air into the lungs. The diaphragm works with muscles of the chest wall, shoulders, and neck to perform ventilation.

Disability: In the Primary Survey, loss, or potential loss of Central Nervous System Function due to brain or spinal-cord injury.

Discharge: Fluid escaping from the site of the infection of inflammation.

Dislocation: Disruption of normal joint anatomy.

Distal: An anatomical direction; away from the body center.

Drowning, near: At least temporary survival of water inhalation. Usually associated with the protective effects of hypothermia in cold water.

Edema: Swelling due to leaking of serum from capillaries.

Epinepherine: The synthetic form of the hormone adrenaline, a vasoconstricting drug.

Evacuation: Removing a patient from the scene of injury or illness, usually enroute to medical care.

Extension: Movement which is the opposite of flexion.

Exudate: Discharge.

Femoral artery: Large artery which travels along the femur in the thigh.

Femur: Long bone of the thigh.

Flail chest: The loss of rigidity of the chest wall due to injury involving multiple fractured ribs.

Flexion: Movement of a joint that brings the extremity closer to the body.

Fracture: Broken bone or cartilage.

Frostbite: Frozen tissue.

Frostnip: Loss of circulation due to the vasoconstriction of blood vessels in the skin during the early stages of tissue freezing.

Glaucoma: Disease or condition causing increased pressure within the globe of the eye.

HACE (High Altitude Cerebral Edema): Swelling of the brain due to oxygen deprivation at high altitude.

Head injury: Injury that involves the brain

Heart attack: An episode of ischemia of heart muscle caused by a blood clot or spasm of the coronary arteries.

Heat challenge: Combined warming effects of humidity, ambient temperature and exercise.

Heat response: The normal body response, including sweating and vasodilation of the shell, to the heat challenge.

Heat stroke: Severe elevation of body temperature (over 105°F).

Hemothorax: Free blood in the chest cavity; usually from injury. (thorax)

Hyperextension: To extend a joint beyond its normal range of motion.

Hyperventilation syndrome: The symptoms caused by reduced carbon dioxide in the blood due to excessive ventilation, usually associated with Acute Stress Reaction.

Hypothermia: Below normal body core temperature (below 96°F). Can be mild (<96°F) or severe (<90°F).

Infection: Invasion of body tissues by bacteria, virus, or other micro-organisms.

Inflammatory process: A generic body response to illness or injury resulting in redness, swelling, warmth, and tenderness.

Intoxicated: Altered Nervous System function due to the influence of chemicals such as drugs, alcohol, and inhaled gasses.

Intracranial: Inside of the skull (cranium).

Ischemia: Lack of local perfusion to body tissues.

IV fluids: Fluids infused directly into the circulatory system through a hypodermic needle inserted into a vein, usually used to temporarily increase the volume of circulating blood.

Ligaments: Tough connective tissue joining bone to bone across joints.

Local effects: Effects which are restricted to the immediate area of injury or infection (versus systematic, total-body effects).

Long bones: Bones which have a long structural axis, such as leg and arm bones, as opposed to flat bones like ribs and shoulder blade.

Lumbar spine: The lower section of the spine between the thorax and the pelvis.

Mechanism of injury: The cause of injury, or the description of the forces involved.

Mental status: Describes the level of brain function in an alert patient (A or AVPU) in terms of memory, level of anxiety, and behavior.

Mid-range position: Position in a joint's range of motion between full extension and full flexion.

Monitor: Regularly repeated patient assessment (SOAP) for the purpose of revising assessments and plans as the situation changes.

Neutral Position: The position approximately half way between flexion and extension.

Open fracture: Fracture with an associated break in the skin.

Oxygenation: To saturate blood with oxygen. Oxygenation of the blood takes place in the lungs.

Patella: Knee cap.

Patient Assessment System: A system of surveys including Scene Survey, Primary Survey, and Secondary Survey, designed to gather information about an injured or ill patient and the environment in which they are found.

Penicillin: An antibiotic drug.

Perfusion: The passage of blood through capillary beds in body tissues.

Peripheral nerves: The nerves running between body tissues and the central nervous system.

Photophobia: Eye pain or headache caused by bright lights.

Pneumonia: Infection of lung tissue.

Pneumothorax: Free air in the chest cavity, usually from a punctured lung or chest wall (thorax). Usually associated with hemothorax.

Primary Survey: The first examination of the injured patient which includes assessment of airway, breathing, circulation, and disability.

Pulmonary edema: Swelling of lung tissue resulting in fluid in the alveoli.

Reduction: Restoring a dislocated joint to normal position. Also restoring a displaced fracture to normal anatomic position.

Scene Survey: The stage of the Patient Assessment System during which you look for dangers to the rescuer and patient, numbers of people injured, and the mechanism of injury.

Secondary Survey: The stage in the Patient Assessment System during which includes the examination of the whole body, AMPLE history, and vital signs.

Seizures: Uncoordinated electrical activity in the brain.

Serum: The liquid portion of the blood, as distinguished from blood cells and platelets.

Sexually Transmitted Disease (STD): Infection generally transmitted from person to person by sexual activity.

Shell/core effect: A compensation mechanism seen in shock and cold response which reduces blood flow to the body shell in order to preserve perfusion and warmth in the vital organs of the core.

Shock: Inadequate perfusion pressure affecting the whole of the body.

Signs: Response elicited by examination, e.g. pain when the examiner touches an injured area (tenderness).

Sinus: Hollow spaces in the bones of the skull.

Sinusitis: Inflammation of the membranous lining of the sinuses, usually due to infection.

Spasm: Involuntary contraction of muscle.

Spinal cord: The cord-like extension of the central nervous system encased within the bones of the spinal column, running from the base of the brain to the mid-lumbar spine.

Spine: The column of body vertebrae extending from the base of the skull to the pelvis.

Stethoscope: An instrument used to transmit body sounds directly to the ears of the examiner via rubber tubes.

Survey: A systematic examination.

Swelling: Increase in fluid in body tissues from bleeding and edema.

Symptoms: Condition described by the patient, e.g. pain on swallowing.

Systemic: Involving the entire body.

Tetanus: A disease caused by toxins released by *Clostridium* *tetani* bacteria which may infect wounds. (Also called lock jaw.)

Thorax: The region of the body between the base of the neck and the top of the abdomen.

Tourniquet: A constricting band used to prevent or restrict the flow of blood to an extremity.

Toxin load: The combined systemic effect of numerous small toxic exposures, ie. a large number of insect bites or man-of-war stings.

Toxins: Chemicals which have a damaging effect on body tissues or the function of the nervous system.

Traction: Tension applied along the long axis of an extremity.

Traction splint: A splint device designed to maintain traction on an extremity, used for femur fractures.

Trauma: Injury.

Trench foot: Inflammation due to the loss of circulation due to constriction of blood vessels in tissues exposed to cold and wet conditions (above freezing) for a prolonged period of time.

Vapor barrier: A wrap or covering which prevents passage of water vapor which reduces the effect of cooling by evaporation.

Vascular bundles: A nerve, artery, and vein following the same pathway.

Vascular shock: Shock due to dilation of blood vessels.

Ventilation: The movement of air in and out of the lungs.

Vertebrae: The bones of the spine.

Vital signs: Measurements of body function including blood pressure, pulse, respiration, consciousness, skin color, and body core temperature.

INDEX